LUNG
CANCER

Dedication

We dedicate this guide to all the relatives and patients that have died fighting lung cancer. Their sacrifice will not be in vain, every day we are getting closer to making lung cancer history.

For Elsevier

Commissioning Editor: Pauline Graham
Development Editor: Barbara Simmons
Project Manager: Susan Stuart
Typesetting and Production: Helius
Designer: George Ajayi

LUNG CANCER

A PRACTICAL GUIDE

Luis E. Raez MD, FACP, FCCP
Associate Professor of Medicine, Epidemiology and Public Health,
Director, Hematology/Oncology Clinics and Chemotherapy Unit (CTU),
Co-Leader Thoracic Oncology Group,
Sylvester Comprehensive Cancer Center,
University of Miami Miller School of Medicine, Florida, USA

Orlando E. Silva MD, JD, FACP, FCLM
Associate Professor of Medicine,
Sylvester Comprehensive Cancer Center,
University of Miami Miller School of Medicine, Florida, USA

EDINBURGH LONDON NEW YORK OXFORD PHILADELPHIA
ST LOUIS SYDNEY TORONTO 2008

SAUNDERS
ELSEVIER

© 2008, Elsevier Limited. All rights reserved.

First published 2008

ISBN: 978-0-7020-2889-2

British Library Cataloguing in Publication Data
A catalogue record for this book is available from the British Library

Library of Congress Cataloging in Publication Data
A catalog record for this book is available from the Library of Congress

Notice
Knowledge and best practice in this field are constantly changing. As new research and experience broaden our knowledge, changes in practice, treatment and drug therapy may become necessary or appropriate. Readers are advised to check the most current information provided (i) on procedures featured or (ii) by the manufacturer of each product to be administered, to verify the recommended dose or formula, the method and duration of administration, and contraindications. It is the responsibility of the practitioner, relying on their own experience and knowledge of the patient, to make diagnoses, to determine dosages and the best treatment for each individual patient, and to take all appropriate safety precautions. To the fullest extent of the law, neither the Publisher nor the Editors assume any liability for any injury and/or damage to persons or property arising out or related to any use of the material contained in this book.   *The Publisher*

Printed in China.

Acknowledgments

The authors would like to thank the following contributing experts for actively participating and offering invaluable advice in the preparation of this handbook. Some helped with the entirety of the book and some with specific chapters as listed under their names.

Carmen Calfa MD
(*Chapter 7*)
Division of Hematology/Oncology,
University of Miami Miller School
of Medicine,
Miami, Florida, USA

Alberto A. Chiappori MD
(*Chapter 11*)
Assistant Professor,
Thoracic Oncology Program,
H. Lee Moffitt Cancer Center and
Research Institute,
Tampa, Florida, USA

**Juan Carlos Hernandez
Umana** MD
(*Chapter 1*)
Division of Hematology/Oncology,
The William Harrington Latin
American Training Program,
University of Miami Miller School
of Medicine,
Miami, Florida, USA

Mohammad Jahanzeb MD, FACP
(*Chapter 10*)
Van Vleet Endowed Professor in
Medical Oncology,
Chief,
Division of Hematology/Oncology,
Fellowship Program Director,
University of Tennessee Health
Science Center,
Memphis, Tennessee, USA

Merce Jorda MD, PhD
(*Chapter 6*)
Associate Professor of Clinical
Pathology,
Medical Director of Laboratory
Services,
Sylvester Comprehensive Cancer
Center,
University of Miami Miller School
of Medicine,
Miami, Florida, USA

Melissa Karr RN, BSN, OCN, RRT
(*Chapters 20, 21*)
Clinical Nurse Coordinator,
Head & Neck and Thoracic
Oncology,
Sylvester Comprehensive Cancer
Center,
University of Miami Miller School
of Medicine,
Miami, Florida, USA

Christian Lobo MD
(*Chapter 17*)
Division of Hematology/Oncology,
University of Miami Miller School
of Medicine,
Miami, Florida, USA

Gilberto Lopez MD
(*Chapter 9*)
Consultant in Oncology,
Johns Hopkins Singapore
International Medical Center,
Johns Hopkins University,
Baltimore, Maryland, USA

Jessica MacIntyre RN, BSN, OCN
(*Chapter 20*)
Pancreatic, Liver and GI Related
Cancers Group,
Sylvester Comprehensive Cancer
Center,
University of Miami Miller School
of Medicine,
Miami, Florida, USA

Daniel Morgensztern MD
(*Chapter 9*)
Instructor,
Department of Medicine,
Division of Medical Oncology,
Washington University School of
Medicine;
Staff Physician,
Division of Hematology/Oncology,
St Louis Veterans Affairs Medical
Center,
St Louis, Missouri, USA

José A. Peñagarícano MD
(*Chapter 14*)
Associate Professor,
Department of Radiation Oncology,
University of Arkansas for
Medical Sciences,
Little Rock, Arkansas, USA

Vaneerat Ratanatharathorn MD, MBA
(*Chapter 14*)
Chair and Professor,

Department of Radiation Oncology,
University of Arkansas for
Medical Sciences,
Little Rock, Arkansas, USA

Caio Max S. Rocha Lima MD
(*Chapters 10, 13*)
Associate Professor of Medicine,
Division of Hematology/Oncology;
Co-Leader Pancreatic, Liver and
Related Cancers Group,
Sylvester Comprehensive Cancer
Center,
University of Miami Miller School
of Medicine,
Miami, Florida, USA

Eloy Roman MD
(*Chapters 8, 15, 21*)
Division of Hematology/Oncology,
University of Miami Miller School
of Medicine,
Miami, Florida, USA

Manuel F. Rosado MD
(*Chapters 7, 12, 16*)
Assistant Professor of Medicine,
Yale University School of
Medicine,
New Haven, Connecticut, USA

Alvaro Daniel Saenz MD
(*Chapter 6*)
Department of Pathology,
St. Anthony's Hospital,
St. Petersburg, Florida, USA

Edgardo S. Santos MD, FACP
(*Chapter 3, 18, 19, 21*)
Assistant Scientific Director,
Office of Clinical Research;
Associate Director,
Hematology/Oncology Fellowship
Program;
Assistant Professor of Medicine,
Division of Hematology–Medical
Oncology,

Tulane University Health
Sciences Center,
New Orleans, Louisiana, USA

Richard J. Thurer MD
(Chapters 7, 12)
B. and Donald Carlin Professor of
Thoracic Surgical Oncology,
Senior Associate Dean for Faculty
Affairs;
Co-Leader,
Thoracic Oncology Group,

Sylvester Comprehensive Cancer
Center,
University of Miami Miller School
of Medicine,
Miami, Florida, USA

Shazia Zafar MD
(Chapter 20)
Division of Hematology/Oncology,
University of Miami Miller School
of Medicine,
Miami, Florida, USA

Foreword

It is with enthusiasm that I introduce you to this exciting book focusing on the management of lung cancer. This book targets a wide audience of busy healthcare professionals who care for patients with lung cancer. The demands on healthcare professionals have increased exponentially. We are faced with a rapid growth of knowledge in all fields of medicine. This phenomenon is no different in the field of oncology. Furthermore, lung cancer imposes this extra burden on practitioners who face critically ill patients daily. This book on lung cancer will assist all healthcare givers caring for patients with lung cancer in their quest of providing the highest possible standard of services to their patients.

The book is not intended to be a comprehensive review of lung cancer, but a 'to the point' reference that one can carry as a pocket book. The chapters are designed to address questions that oncology care providers face constantly. The chapters are purposely short, brief, and concise. The important facts are presented as bullet points, emphasizing the relevant aspects of the topic of the chapter. The busy reader will be able to cruise through the information effortlessly. References are provided so that one can expand on the topic being addressed.

It is not the intention of this book to replace well-establish oncology guidelines and books. It is suggested that readers consult well-established sources of information, such as the National Comprehensive Cancer Network (NCCN), American College of Chest Physicians (ACCP), or American Society of Clinical Oncology (ASCO) guidelines, among others. However, the information provided in this book will help with the decision-making process for most cases of lung cancer seen in our practices. However, the authors do not want to disappoint readers who hope to find something challenging and new. The topics of immuno-therapy, methylation, and epidermal growth factor (EGFR) inhibitors, and their relevance in lung cancer are addressed.

I invite you to make this book a companion in your busy daily practice. Dr Raez and Dr Silva, whom I know personally and consider good friends, and admire as outstanding oncologists, have put their hearts into compiling this excellent piece of work. I am sure you will enjoy consulting this manual and take advantage of its great value.

Caio Max S. Rocha Lima MD
Associate Professor of Medicine,
Co-Leader Phase I Program, and
Pancreatic, Liver and Related Cancers Group,
Sylvester Comprehensive Cancer Center,
University of Miami Miller School of Medicine,
Miami, Florida, USA

How to use this book

This handbook is written to be a 'bedside' reference for oncologists of the various specialties, as well as a compendium of lung cancer information useful to thoracic surgeons, pulmonologists, respiratory medicine specialists, clinical researchers and educators, medical students, and nurses.

This is a small book, and it was never intended to be a comprehensive textbook. It is a guide for busy oncology fellows, general oncologists, and other healthcare professionals who need a rapid and succinct review of the basic information. We invite everybody to take some time and review the references of the specific topic that is of interest to you. The text is written telegraphically, in outline format, emphasizing the key concepts. By this means, the reader has an immediately accessible portal to the current literature, the major trials, the landmark articles, and the reviews up to the time of writing this book. The results of important trials are summarized in 5–10 lines, with key data including: whether or not randomized, number of subjects, study period, median follow-up, doses, results, limitations and conclusions. In addition, there is a comprehensive index, so that specific information can be found quickly.

We quote the most important references, sometimes including doses and schemas of administration of anticancer agents. However, due to the fast evolving pace of anticancer research, we strongly recommend readers to check the latest labels of all oncology products referred to in this book, and to review latest developments in the field before treating patients.

It is our hope that this compendium will be not only an aid to the physician involved in patient care, but also to physician scientists, as it indicates where knowledge is lacking and understanding is incomplete, and thus suggests targets for future research. We plan to continue publishing periodic updates as progress in combating this major health problem continues.

Commonly used abbreviations

ACORN	American Clinical Oncology Research Network	ECOG	Eastern Cooperative Oncology Group
ALPI	Adjuvant Lung Project Italy	ED-SCLC	Extensive-disease, small-cell lung cancer
ANITA	Adjuvant Navelbine International Trialist Association	EGFR	Epidermal growth factor
		ELCAP	Early Lung Cancer Action Project
ARR	Absolute risk reduction		
ASCO	American Society of Clinical Oncology	ELISA	Enzyme-linked immunosorbent assay
ATP	Adenosine 5′-triphosphate	ELVIS	Elderly Lung Cancer Vinorelbine Italian Study
ATS	American Thoracic Society		
AUC	Area under the curve	EORTC	European Organization for Research and Treatment of Cancer
BAC	Bronchioalveolar carcinoma		
BALT	Bronchus-associated lymphoid tissue	EPP	Extrapleural pneumonectomy
BCG	Bacillus Calmette–Guerin	ER	Estrogen receptor
BLOT	Bimodality Lung Oncology Team	ETS	Environmental tobacco smoke
		EUS FNA	Esophageal, endoscopic, ultrasound-guided, fine needle aspiration
BLT	Big Lung Trial		
BSC	Best supportive care		
CALG	Cancer and Leukemia Group	EUS TCB	Esophageal, endoscopic, ultrasound-guided, trucut biopsy
CALGB	Cancer and Leukemia Group B		
CEA	Carcinoembryonic antigen		
cfu	Colony-forming unit	FACS	Four-Arm Cooperative Study
CINV	Chemotherapy-induced nausea and vomiting	FDA	Food and Drug Administration (USA)
CNS	Central nervous system	FDG	[^{18}F]Deoxyglucose
COX-2	Cyclooxygenase-2	FHIT	Fragile histidine triad
CR	Complete response	FNA	Fine needle aspiration
CT	Computerized tomography	FTI	Farnesyltransferase inhibitor
CTL	Cytotoxic T-lymphocyte	GAR	Good antibody responder
DC	Dendritic cell	GCSF	Granulocyte colony-stimulating factor
DFS	Disease-free survival		
DHAC	Dihydro-5-azacytidine	GM-CSF	Granulocyte–macrophage colony-stimulating factor
DLT	Dose-limiting toxicity		
EBUS	Endobronchial, ultrasound-guided, needle aspirate	GRPR	Gastrin-releasing peptide receptor

HDAC	Histone deacetylase	PCR	Polymerase chain reaction
HIV	Human immunodeficiency virus	PD	Progression of disease
		PDT	Photodynamic therapy
HPF	High-power field	PET	Positron emission tomography
HPV	Human papilloma virus	PFS	Progression-free survival
HR	Hazard ratio	p.o.	By mouth
IALT	International Adjuvant Lung Cancer Trial	PR	Progesterone receptor
		PR	Partial response
IARC	International Agency for Research on Cancer	PS	Performance status
		PTT	Prothombin time
IL-10	Interleukin-10	q	Every
INR	International normalized ratio	QOL	Quality of life
INTACT	Iressa NSCLC Trial Assessing Combination Trial	RAR	Retinoic acid receptor
		RARE	Retinoic acid response element
ISEL	Iressa Survival Evaluation in Lung Cancer	RDOG	Radiologic Diagnostic Oncologic Group
IU	International units	RECIST	Response Evaluation Criteria in Solid Tumors
i.v.	Intravenous		
KHL	Keyhole limpet hemocyanin	RFA	Radiofrequency ablation
LCSG	Lung Cancer Study Group	RFS	Relapse-free survival
LD-SCLC	Limited-disease small-cell lung cancer	ROC	Receiver operating characteristic
LN	Lymph node	RR	Response rate
LVI	Lymphovascular invasion	RR	Relative risk
MAPK	Mitogen-activated protein kinase	RRR	Relative risk of recurrence
		RTOG	Radiation Therapy Oncology Group
MILES	Multicenter Italian Lung Cancer in the Elderly Study	RXR	Retinoid X receptor
ml	Milliliter	s.c.	Subcutaneous
MLND	Mediastinal lymph node dissection	SCC	Squamous cell carcinoma
		SCLC	Small-cell lung cancer
MM	Malignant mesothelioma	SD	Stable disease
MRI	Magnetic resonance imaging	SECSG	Southeastern Cancer Study Group
MSKCC	Memorial Sloan Kettering Cancer Center	SEER	Surveillance, Epidemiology, and End Results
MTD	Maximum tolerated dose	SICOG	Southern Italy Cooperative Group
NADH	Nicotinamide adenine dinucleotide		
NCI	National Cancer Institute	SPN	Solitary pulmonary nodule
NCCN	National Comprehensive Cancer Network	SUR	Standardized uptake ratio
		SWOG	Southwest Oncology Group
NS	Not significant	TBNA	Transbronchial needle aspiration
NSCLC	Non-small-cell lung cancer		
NSCLCCG	Non-Small-Cell Lung Cancer Collaborative Group	TK	Tyrosine kinase
		TKI	Tyrosine kinase inhibitor
OR	Odds ratio	TTNA	Transthoracic needle aspiration
ORR	Overall response rate		
OS	Overall survival	TTP	Time to progression
PCI	Prophylactic cranial irradiation	VATS	Video-assisted thoracocoscopy

VEGF	Vascular endothelial growth factor	CV	Cisplatin + vindesine
vs	Versus, or compared to	DDP	Cisplatin
WBC	White blood count	EP	Etoposide + cisplatin
WHO	World Health Organization	MIC	Mitomycin + ifosfamide + cisplatin
XRT	Radiation therapy	MIP	Mitomycin + ifosfamide + cisplatin
♀	Woman or female		
♂	Man or male	MVP	Mitomycin + vinblastine + cisplatin

Drugs and drug combinations

5-FU	5-Fluorouracil	NP	Vinorelbine + cisplatin
CAMP	Cytophosphamide + adriamycin + methotrexate + procarbazine	PCV	Cisplatin + cyclophosphamide + vindesine
CAV	Cyclophosphamide + doxorubicin + vincristine	PET	Cisplatin + paclitaxel + etoposide
CAV	Cytoxan + Adriamycin + vincristine	TEP	Paclitaxel + etoposide + cisplatin
CEV	Cyclophosphamide + epirubicin + vincristine		

Drug combinations are defined on first usage within a chapter.

Contents

Contents

Contents

History of lung cancer

[Onuigbo WIB, Lung cancer in the nineteenth century, Med Hist 3(1): 69–77, 1959]
[Onuigbo WIB, Historical notes on cancer, Med Hist 2(2): 114–119, 1958]
[Ackerknecht EH, Historical trends in cancer surgery, Med Hist 6: 154–161, 1962]
[Rosenblatt MB, Lung cancer, Bull Hist Med 38: 395–425, 1964]

3400 BC to 1774 AD

- Paleopathological evidence (bone evidence) of cancer has been found in cave bears and Pleistocene horses.

- 3400 BC: Osteosarcomata in Egyptian skulls from the first (3400 BC) and fifth (c. 2750 BC) dynasties have been described.

- 1500 BC: 'swellings' and 'ulcers' of skin, mamma and female genitalia described in Egyptian papyri. They were treated by excision or caustic salves, just as today. The same descriptions are encountered in ancient medical writings from Mesopotamia, India and Persia.

- 400 BC: Hippocrates wrote: 'Where non-inflammatory hard swelling and ulcers of the skin, female breast and genitalia with tendency to generalization, recidive and fatal ending are described under the names of karkinos or karkarkinoma', translated into Latin as 'cancer'.

- 150 AD: The great physician Galen wrote a special book of 'tumours'. He described edema and erysipelas as well as lipoma and cancer.

- Early observations by Agricola (1527) and Van Swieten (1747) described lung cancer resembling brain tissue, using terms such as 'encephaloid' and 'cerebriform'. Agricola went further, identifying lung cancer as an endemic occupational disease in miners from Saxony and Bohemia.

- 1757: The French surgeon Le Dran was the first to try transplantation of cancerous tissue into an animal, the dog.

1775 to 1900

[Onuigbo WIB, Lung cancer in the nineteenth century, Med Hist **3**(1): 69–77, 1959]
[Onuigbo WIB, Historical notes on cancer, Med Hist **2**(2): 114–119, 1958]

- 1775: Pott illustrated the association between chimney sweepers and scrotal cancer as well as pulmonary cancer (1879).

- 1810: Bayle reported the first case of Primary lung cancer. 'A 72-year-old patient with cough, white expectoration, lack of appetite, liver enlarged and three indolent, movable bodies, about the size of nuts, found in the epigastric and hypochondriac region. The patient dies and the necropsy showed: a mass of shining, white appearance, which resembles the brain. The liver contained numerous cerebriform masses, and the movable, subcutaneous bodies were evidently of the same nature as the internal tumor.'

- 1815: Laenec differentiated the so-called 'cerebriform/encephaloid' lesion from tuberculosis. The word 'encephaloid,' from the Greek *Enkephalos*, means resembling the brain or brain tissue (cancer of soft, brain like consistency).

- 1819: According to Dr Cockle (1865), Dr Baron was the first to diagnose lung cancer in living person.

Etiology

[Onuigbo WIB, Lung cancer in the nineteenth century, Med Hist **3**(1): 69–77, 1959]

- 1875: Loomis and Ingals (1892) attributed lung cancer to diathesis; in general they found that men were affected more often than women, the incidence being mainly between 40 and 60 years of age.

- 1878: Hesse wrote a paper in which he drew attention to the high incidence of lung cancer among miners in Schneeberg, Germany.

This was corroborated by Osler in 1892: 'it is remarkable that the workers in the Schneeberg cobalt mines are very liable to primary cancer of the lungs'.

Clinical features

[Onuigbo WIB, Lung cancer in the nineteenth century, *Med Hist* **3**(1): 69–77, 1959]

- 1842: Stokes emphasized the need for vigilance whenever 'we see a patient attacked with severe symptoms of pulmonary disease which resist ordinary treatment'. He knew that in cancer of the lung the accompanying signs of irritation are observed to be influenced by treatment or, if they were removed, they return again and again without apparent cause.

- 1843: Greene reported the presence of extrapulmonary symptoms. Not infrequently, they are cerebral. He also observed that deposits deep in the frontal lobes did not give rise to pain.

- 1848: Blakinston case report: Active treatment also failed to make any impression on the disease, and the trachea and esophagus were seen to be gradually compressed.

- 1865: Cockle wrote an early monograph on intrathoracic growths. He made the point that 'brain deposits and irritation of the meninges play an important part in the clinical history of thoracic cancer'. He was clear when he said that 'disturbed cerebral function so frequently coexists with intrathoracic cancer'.

- 1839: John Reid reported a single case of an unknown syndrome which was later attributed to Horner himself (1869). In fact, William Gairdner and Argyll Robertson accepted this to be John Reid's own discovery.

Diagnosis

[Onuigbo WIB, Lung cancer in the nineteenth century, *Med Hist* **3**(1): 69–77, 1959]

- 1837: Stokes published different papers related with the diagnosis of lung cancer: 'Aneurism, circumscribed pleuritic effusion, and enlargement of the heart; pleuropnuemonia, pleurisy, and hepatization, in consequence of previous pneumonia; solidification from tuberculosis. I gave up all further attempts at diagnosis.'

- 1853: Skoda illustrated the use of the stethoscope as a tool in the diagnoses of lung cancer: 'percussion is helpful when the encephaloid disease of the pleura is considerably extended'.

- 1846: Addison indicated that percussion and auscultation are insufficient for the diagnoses of lung cancer, adding that paracentesis was, on occasion, diagnostic.

- 1866: Austin Flints: 'It is possible that microscopical characters of cancer may be discovered in the sputa.'

- 1898: Hampeln concluded that there are many details of size, shape, character of the nucleus, and stating properties that, when considered in relation to their source, may enable an experienced observer to draw conclusions of value.

- 1895: Kirstein was the first to obtain a direct view of the vocal cords and the forking of the trachea. It was the beginning of the laryngoscopy and bronchoscopy.

- The last decade of the nineteenth century witnessed the advent of radiography.

Pathology

[Onuigbo WIB, Lung cancer in the nineteenth century, *Med Hist* 3(1): 69–77, 1959]

- 1857: Orr reported details of lung necropsy in patients with lung malignancy.

- 1880: Bartholow reported tumor involvement to be mostly in the right lung.

- 1888: Byrom Bramwell and Risien Rusell (1899) held that bronchial carcinomas were the most common source of intracranial metastasis. Later, Strumpell (1893) said that breast cancer shared this notoriety with lung cancer.

- 1889: Hanford illustrated the metastasis of lung cancer to the liver and kidney.

- 1891: Fox described lymph node metastasis and noted the spread, usually centrifugal, to adjoining nodes.

- 1892: Gazayerly and others believed that growths arose in the lymph node and only later invaded the bronchus: 'They originated in the lymphatic tissue at the root of the lung, and only affected the lung by direct extension.'

- In the succeeding decades this area was moved forward, notably by James Paget (1853), Virchow (1860), Campbell De Morgan (1874), Augustus Pepper (1884) and Coats (1895).

Treatment and prognosis

[Onuigbo WIB, Historical notes on cancer, Med Hist 2(2): 114–119, 1958] [Ackerknecht EH, Historical trends in cancer surgery, Med Hist 6: 154–161, 1962]

- 1895: Sir William Macenwen used cauterization to evacuate necrotic tissue from a patient with tuberculosis.

- 1896: Stephen Paget said: 'The most that can be done, and, so far as we can see, that ever will be done, is to withdraw the effusion'.

1900 to 2000

[Onuigbo WIB, Historical notes on cancer, Med Hist 2(2): 114–119, 1958] [Rosenblatt MB, Lung cancer, Bull Hist Med 38: 395–425, 1964]

- 1912: Adler reported cigarette smoking as on etiologic factor of lung cancer.
  - However, it was not until 1952 that Doll and Hill clearly demonstrated the strong epidemiological association between cigarette smoking and lung cancer.

- 1922: Lillienthal reported 22 lobectomies with a 42% mortality rate.

- 1931: The first two-step pneumonectomy was done in Germany by Nissen.

- 1933: The first one-stage total pneumonectomy was performed in the USA by Dr Graham, who operated on Dr Gilmore, a 48-year-old obstetrician who had undifferentiated squamous cell carcinoma of the left upper lung.

- 1930–1980: The incidence of lung cancer increased dramatically, from 956 reported cases in 1930 to 87 per 100,000 individuals by 1984.

- 1948: Karnofsky reported the first series of patients treated with nitrogen mustard for lung carcinoma.

- 1960: The first randomized trial of chemotherapy agents
  - Thiophosphoramide vs nitrogen mustard.
  - Reported a higher objective response for nitrogen mustard, but no significant survival difference.

- 1974: Rosemberg and colleagues used cisplatin for patients with testicular cancer.
  - Response rates $\rightarrow$ 20% to 30%.
  - Later it was used to treat lung cancer.
  - Lung Cancer Collaborative Group (1995) favored cisplatin-containing chemotherapy.

- 1990: New, well-tolerated drugs developed, including vinorelbine, gemcitabine, docetaxel and paclitaxel.

- 2003–2004: First tyrosine kinase inhibitors (TKI), gefinitib and erlotinib, were approved for use in lung cancer, starting the era of 'targeted therapy' in lung cancer.

- 2004: Pemetrexed, an antifolate, was approved for patients with non-small-cell lung cancer who had failed on first-line chemotherapy.
  - The drug has a better toxicity profile than other chemotherapeutic agents, in particular a lower rate of neutropenia.

- 2005: Advances in anti-angiogenesis led to an improvement of therapy against lung cancer with the recombinant anti-VEGF antibody bevacizumab.

2

Epidemiology of lung cancer

- The high incidence of lung cancer and the poor survival rate make lung cancer a very important public health problem and the leading cause of cancer death in the world.

Risk factors associated with lung cancer

- There is no doubt that tobacco is the single most important risk factor.
  - There are other important factors, and there are still a number of lung cancers for which the etiologies are unknown.

- Cigarette smoking is the single most predominant cause of the lung cancer epidemic.
  [Alberg A, *J Clin Oncol* **23**(14): 3175–3185, 2005]
  - Other contributing agents are: asbestos, arsenic, chromium, nickel, radon, and other environmental factors, such as passive smoking and air pollution.

- Lung cancer accounts for 12% of all cancers diagnosed worldwide, making it the most common malignancy, other than skin cancer.
  [World Health Organization, International Agency for Research on Cancer (IARC). *World Cancer Report*. Lyon, France, IARC Press, 2003]

- Since the release of the 1964 report from the US Surgeon General, we know that smoking causes lung cancer in ♂; it took more years to reach the same conclusion in ♀.

[US Department of Health Education and Welfare. *Smoking and Health*. Report of the Advisory Committee to the Surgeon General. DHEW Publication No. [PHS] 1103. Washington, DC, US Government Printing Office, 1964]

- Lung cancer tends to be most common in developed countries, particularly in North America and Europe, and less common in developing countries, particularly in Africa and South America.
  [Pisani P, *Int J Cancer* **83**: 18–29, 1999]
  - In all countries the rates of lung cancer are higher in ♂, which is probably related to historic patterns of smoking.
    [Khuder SA, *Lung Cancer* **31**: 139–148, 2000]

- In the initial decades of the smoking-caused epidemic of lung cancer, squamous cell carcinoma was the most frequent type of lung cancer observed among smokers, and small-cell carcinoma was the next most frequent.
  [US Department of Health and Human Services. *Women and Smoking*. A report of the Surgeon General. Rockville, MD, US Department of Health and Human Services, 2001]
  - After steadily ↑ occurrence during 1973–1987, adenocarcinoma became the most frequent form of lung cancer.

- Smoking causes each of the major histologic types of lung cancer, although the trend in risk with number of cigarettes smoked varies across the types, being steepest for small-cell undifferentiated carcinoma.

[Bek K, *Postgrad Med J* **75**: 339–341, 1999]
[Cunningham J, *Am J Respir Crit Care Med* **153**: 218–224, 1996]
[Farkas AJ, *Prev Med* **28**: 213–218, 1999]
[Mannino DM, *Chest* **122**: 409–415, 2002]

- Children who are exposed to environmental tobacco smoke (ETS) are at ↑ risk of asthma, respiratory infections, and premature death.

- The severity of respiratory tract disease ↑ in accordance with degree of exposure.

- Parents who smoke put children and spouses at risk for adverse health outcomes, and ↑ the chance that their children will become smokers.

- Both the American Academy of Pediatrics and the American Academy of Family Physicians advise that parents should be counseled as to the adverse effects of ETS on child health.

- There are reports of the association of small-cell lung cancer in excess in workers exposed to chloromethyl ethers and in underground miners exposed to radon.
  [National Research Council: Committee on Health Risks of Exposure to Radon, Board on Radiation Effects Research, and Commission on Life Sciences. *Health Effects of Exposure to Radon* (BEIR VI). Washington, DC, National Academy Press, 1998]

- There is interest in finding an association between the use of illicit drugs, such as marijuana, and lung cancer.
  [Barsky SH, *Alcohol* **35**(3): 265–275, 2005]
  - There are only reports with small numbers of patients. There is no definite evidence that this link exists.

Lung cancer and race and ethnicity

[US Cancer Statistics Working Group. *United States Cancer Statistics: 2001 Incidence and Mortality.* Atlanta, GA, US Department of Health and Human Services, Centers for Disease Control and Prevention, and National Cancer Institute, 2004]

- This is a controversial topic and deserves a special section.

- Several studies report differences in lung cancer incidence and mortality.
  - It is not clear if these differences can be explained solely by socio-economic problems and poor access to healthcare.

- The National Cancer Institute's Surveillance, Epidemiology, and End Results (SEER) Program and the Centers for Disease Control and Prevention's National Program of Cancer Registries (NPCR) in the third report on nationwide cancer incidence in 2001 mentions a 26% difference in lung cancer incidence rates between black and white ♂ (109.0 to 86.8 per 100,000 per year) in the NPCR/SEER data and 36% in the SEER data alone for the period 1997–2001 (104.1 to 76.6 per 100,000 per year).

- The higher mortality rates of lung cancer in black Americans compared to white Americans can be attributed not only to higher incidence rates, but also to the poorer survival of lung cancer patients who are black compared with those who are white.
  - This racial gap persists within each stage at diagnosis, and for ♂ and ♀.

- Do black Americans get the same access to healthcare; and, if so, will their outcome be the same?
  - This remains to be determined.

- Lung cancer mortality rates among Hispanics, Native Americans, and Asians/Pacific Islanders are significantly lower than the mortality rates among blacks and non-Hispanic whites.
  - Nevertheless, lung cancer poses a considerable public health burden among these groups.
    [National Cancer Institute. *Cancer Rates and Risks*. National Cancer Institute, Bethesda, MD, 2004]

- There is a consensus that lung cancer is more likely to occur in the poor and the less educated.
  [Mao Y, *Int J Epidemiol* **30**: 809–817, 2001]
  [Li K, *J Environ Sci Health C, Environ Carcinogen Ecotoxicol Rev* **20**: 21–28, 2002]
  - A pattern that is observed in many countries worldwide even after adjustment for cigarette smoking.

- In China, those classified as having low income had a six-fold ↑ risk of lung cancer compared with those in the high income category.

Chemoprevention and lung cancer

[Alberg AJ, *Encyclopedia of Human Nutrition*. London, Academic Press, 235–248, 1998]

- Results of chemoprevention trials failed to show that β-carotene, α-tocopherol, or retinol protect against lung cancer in high-risk groups.

- Results of case–control and prospective cohort studies have shown that individuals with a high dietary intake of fruits or vegetables have a lower risk of lung cancer.

Molecular changes associated with lung cancer development

- Several molecular changes in lung cancer have been studied, and there are ongoing investigations to determine their exact role, prognostic relevance, and possible use as therapeutic targets.

Methylation, smoking, and lung cancer

[Belinsky SA, *Cancer Res* **62**: 2370–2377, 2002]
[Swafford DS, *Mol Cell Biol* **17**: 1366–1374, 1997]
[Toyooka S, *Int J Cancer* **110**: 462–464, 2004]
[Tomizawa Y, *Lung Cancer* **46**: 305–312, 2004]

- Smokers without lung cancer had a 35% frequency of p16 promoter hypermethylation in their sputum, but methylation was not detected in the bronchial epithelium of never-smokers.

- Smoking produces an ↑ in epigenetic and genetic changes over time, with ↑ changes with greater amount smoked.
  - RARβ was methylated more frequently in people with a smoking history than in never-smokers.
  - Moreover, the frequency of RARβ methylation ↑ with the severity of the clinical stage of the lung cancer.

- p16, the tumor suppressor gene, is a frequent target for inactivation in lung cancer by epigenetic silencing or genetic deletions.

- Lung cancer in smokers with a < 30 pack-year history had significantly less frequent p16 and RASSF1A methylation than lung cancers in smokers with a > 30 pack-year history, with a dose–response relationship reported.

K-ras, p53, and other changes in lung cancer

[Rodenhuis S, *Cancer Res* **52**: 2665s–2669s, 1992]
[Slebos RJ, *J Natl Cancer Inst* **83**: 1024–1027, 1991]

- Mutations of the *H-*, *K-*, and *N-ras* family of oncogenes are common in lung cancer.

- The *K-ras* gene is the most often mutated, with point mutations occurring predominately at codon 12 and, occasionally, at codons 13 or 61.
  - These mutations result in amino acid substitutions that preserve the activated conformation of *K-ras*, leading to constitutively functioning signal transduction and uncontrolled cell proliferation.
  - *K-ras* mutation is particularly common in patients with an extensive smoking history, with prevalences of approximately 30% vs 5% in pulmonary adenocarcinomas compared with non-smokers.

- *p53* is abnormal in *c.* 50% of non-small-cell lung cancers and 90% of small-cell lung tumors.
  [D'Amico D, *Oncogene* **7**: 339–346, 1992]
  - The *p53* gene encodes for a 53-kDa nuclear phosphoprotein that directs the cells to arrest either at the GI/S or the G2/mitosis phase if the cell suffers DNA damage.
  - Alternatively, *p53* induces the cell towards an apoptotic death.
    [Wistuba II, *Cancer Res* **59**: 1973–1979, 1999]

- One of the most consistent abnormalities in lung cancer is the loss or inactivation of genetic material on the short arm of chromosome 3 (3p).
  - Even in lung cancer patients with 3p changes detectable in tumor, > 30% of non-malignant bronchial epithelium also had 3p changes.

Tyrosine kinase inhibitors and lung cancer

[Lynch TJ, *N Engl J Med* **350**: 2129–2139, 2004]
[Huang SF, *Clin Cancer Res* **10**: 8195–8203, 2004]

- Seem more effective in non-smokers, ♀, young, with an adenocarcinoma, and of Asian ethnicity.

- Further investigations have shown that these populations seem to have not only mutations in the tyrosine kinase inhibitor (TKI) domain, but also larger amounts of EGFR gene (demonstrated by fluorescence in situ hybridization (FISH)).

- Multivariate analysis has so far demonstrated only that survival is associated with multiple gene copies in patients with bronchoalveolar carcinoma.
  [Hirsch F, *Proc Am Soc Clin Oncol* **23**(Suppl a): 7030, 2005]

Screening for lung cancer

[Ellis SM, *Clin Radiol* **56**: 691–699, 2001]
[Landis SH, CA *Cancer J Clin* **48**: 6–29, 1998]
[Hulka BS, *Cancer* **62**(Suppl): 1776–1780, 1988]
[US Preventive Services Task Force. *Guide to Clinical Preventive Services*. Baltimore, MD, Williams & Wilkins, 1989]

- The interest in lung cancer screening is renewed.

- The failure to demonstrate a reduction in mortality in previous lung cancer screening trials, based on chest radiography, led to the widely held conclusion that screening for lung cancer is ineffective.

- Lung cancer, the most common cause of death from malignancy, owed its poor prognosis to the late stage at which the disease was diagnosed.

- The prognosis of early stages, which are usually asymptomatic, is more favorable, especially in non-small-cell histologic types.
  - Consequently, early detection using new imaging techniques promises a reduction in mortality from lung cancer.

- Screening is performed to detect disease at a stage when cure or control is possible.
  - It presumes that a test or series of tests will identify asymptomatic persons at risk of a specific disease.
  - If a patient has a positive screening test, early diagnosis can be made, and consequently a prompt therapeutic intervention, resulting in decreased mortality (the number of disease-specific deaths relative to the total number of persons evaluated).

- At present, screening for early detection of lung cancer is not recommended, probably because of the failure of early studies to demonstrate any mortality reduction from lung cancer evaluations based on sputum cytology and/or chest radiography.
  - With the introduction of helical computerized tomography (CT), a new imaging modality that can detect nodules as small as a few millimeters, the potential benefits of lung cancer screening are being re-examined.

Non-imaging methods for lung cancer screening

[Tockman MS, *Clin Cancer Res* **3**: 2237–2246, 1997]
[Fong KM, *J Thorac Cardiovasc Surg* **118**: 1136–1152, 1999]
[Crowell RE, *Cancer Epidemiol Biomarker Prev* **5**: 631–637, 1996]
[Lam S, *Chest* **113**: 696–702, 1998]
[Ikeda N, *Lung Cancer* **19**: 161–166, 1998]
[Patz EF, *N Engl J Med* **343**: 1627–1633, 2000]
[Szabo E, *Semin Oncol* **20**: 374–382, 1993]
[Lam S, *Clin Chest Med* **20**: 53–61, 1999]
[Mulshine JL, *Hematol Oncol Clin North Am* **11**: 235–252, 1997]
[Jacobson DR, *Ann Oncol* **6**(Suppl 3): S3–S8, 1995]
[Swisher SG, *J Natl Cancer Inst* **91**: 763–771, 1999]
[Pilotti S, *Acta Cytol* **26**: 649–654, 1982]
[Tockman MS, *Chest* **106**(60 Suppl): 385S–390S, 1994]

- The non-imaging methods for early detection have not been tested as the sole method of detection in large trials.
  - Previous screening trials using cytologic sputum examination failed to show a ↓ in disease-specific mortality.

- Sputum samples, bronchoalveolar-lavage fluid, and bronchial-biopsy specimens have been analyzed for findings associated with neoplasia (abnormal patterns of immunostaining, malignant changes, genetic mutations (e.g. in p53 and K-ras), telomerase activity, microsatellite instability, and abnormal DNA methylation).
  - The sensitivity and specificity of tests remain suboptimal.

- Knowledge of the molecular events during the early stages of lung cancer, such as changes in the expression of the fragile histidine triad (FHIT) gene and the presence in sputum of cells with genetic abnormalities, offers possibilities for early diagnosis for former smokers and those who continue to smoke.

- The routine use of annual sputum examination for cytologic assessment is not cost-effective in the detection of early lung cancer.
  - Dysplastic changes identified at sputum cytology, however, should be followed up.
  - There is a possible development of a monoclonal antibody that may improve the yearly detection rate of lung cancer using specific monoclonal antibodies.

Imaging methods for lung cancer screening

[Patz EF, *N Engl J Med* **343**: 1627–1633, 2000]
[Henschke CI, *Ann N Y Acad Sci* **952**: 124–134, 2001]
[Strauss GM, *Chest* **111**: 754–768, 1997]
[Midthun DE, **19**: 59–70, 1998]
[Strauss GM, *Surg Oncol Clin N Am* **8**: 371–387, 1999]
[Berlin NI, *Am Rev Respir Dis* **130**: 565–567, 1984]
[Berlin NI, *Am Rev Respir Dis* **130**: 545–549, 1984]

- In the 1950s, four non-randomized, uncontrolled screening studies (the Philadelphia Pulmonary Neoplasm Research Project, the Veterans Administration Trial, the Tokyo Metropolitan Government Study, and the South London Lung Cancer Study) were reviewed.
  - These studies showed no benefit from screening using chest radiography.

- The North London Cancer Study in 1959 and the Erfurt County Study in 1972, both non-randomized-controlled trials, showed an increase in the number of cancers that could be resected and higher survival rates.
  - Nevertheless, neither trial showed a clear reduction in mortality from lung cancer in the screened groups compared with controls.

- In the 1970s, the Johns Hopkins Lung Project, the Memorial Sloan-Kettering Lung Project, the Mayo Lung Project, and the Czechoslovakian Study (randomized, controlled trials) demonstrated a statistically significant difference between the screened and control groups in mortality attributable to lung cancer.

- The National Cancer Institute (NCI) Cooperative Early Lung Cancer Group screened 30,000 high-risk ♂ volunteers (e.g. ♂ cigarette smokers aged > 45 years).
  - Lung cancers identified by screening methods were more frequently early-stage tumors (40% vs 15%) in the high-risk group than in the control group.

- Lung cancer 5-year survival was 35% in the screened group compared with 13% in the general population.
- The same results were obtained in Europe, where mass screening for lung cancer by chest radiography or sputum cytology (or both) cannot be recommended.
- CONCLUSION:
  - Screening had no impact on overall survival in the two groups when all deaths were considered.

- In 1993, the Early Lung Cancer Action Project (ELCAP) initiated and experimentally screened a cohort of 1,000 high-risk subjects.
  - The study consisted of a baseline and annual repeated CT screening of the 1,000 subjects.
  - RESULTS:
    - The study confirmed that CT is more sensitive than conventional chest radiography for the detection of lung nodules and that some of these nodules prove to be lung cancer.

[Ohmatsu H, *Proc Am Soc Clin Oncol* **18**: 1787 (abstract), 1999]
[Henschke CI, *Lancet* **354**: 99–105, 1999]
[Flehinger BJ, *Chest* **101**: 1013–1018, 1992]
- A significant number of very early primary tumors have been identified using low-dose spiral CT with significantly improved 5-year survival outcome in treated patients.
  - The use of low-dose spiral CT scans has confirmed the ability to discover extremely early lung cancers, with a prevalence rate of 30 per 1000 (vs 3000–4000 with plain chest radiographs).
  - Whether the discovery of early treatable cancers ultimately affects the overall long-term mortality in a mass screening population will have to be determined prospectively.
  - The 5-year survival of screen-detected stage I lung cancer falls from nearly 70% to less than 20% if left untreated, suggesting a significant benefit from earlier treatment.

[Strauss GM, *J Clin Oncol* **20**(8): 1973–1983, 2002]
- A regression analysis was performed in this study, which has been interpreted as negative because it failed to demonstrate a mortality reduction among those subjects randomized to chest radiography and cytology.
  - In contrast, the survival suggested that screening was highly effective.
  - The study included 9,192 patients.
  - The conclusion drawn from this analysis was that survival was superior in the screened population, and this advantage was not

attributable to lead-time bias, length bias, or overdiagnosis bias. Mortality was biased, because incidence differences confounded the ability of mortality to reflect the true effect of screening.

Cost-effectiveness in lung cancer screening.

[Marshall D, *Eur J Cancer* **37**: 1759–1767, 2001]
[National Cancer Institute, *Surveillance, Epidemiology, and End Results (SEER) Cancer Statistics Review*, 1973–1997]

- Several features of lung cancer suggest it may be a good candidate for screening.
  - High mortality rate.
  - Difference in survival by stage of disease.
  - Current low rate of early detection.
  - Availability of early intervention for early detection.
  - High cost of advanced disease.

- According to estimates from the SEER (Surveillance, Epidemiology and End Results) registry, the overall 5-year survival rate for patients diagnosed with lung cancer is approximately 14% in the USA.
  - If surgical intervention is performed, the 5-year survival rate improves to 60–70% for patients with stage I lung cancer, and is as high as 70–80% for patients with very early disease.
  - These observations suggest that early detection in a screening program will result in very good prognosis.

- This study (model developed from ELCAP data; observational cohort and not a randomized controlled trial) found that for a cohort of very high-risk patients aged 60–74 years, annual screening for lung cancer over a period of 5 years appears to be cost-effective at $18,968/life-year saved.
  - With a 1-year decrease in survival benefit incorporated in the model, annual screening remained cost-effective at $61,723/life-year saved.
  - The result of this study was consistent with those performed at the H. Lee Moffitt Cancer Center at the University of South Florida.

- Both model predictions for lung cancer screening are within the range of estimates for colorectal cancer screening, mammography screening (♀ aged 45–69 years), and hypertension screening, and are well below those for prostate cancer screening and annual mammography for ♀ aged 40–49 years.

- In summary, the promising results from ELCAP have created speculation that screening for lung cancer using low-dose, helical CT might have a dramatic impact on lung cancer mortality.
  - However, there is insufficient evidence to recommend routine population screening for lung cancer.
  - Well-designed, randomized, controlled trials are necessary to clarify this question.

Ongoing trials

- A prospective, randomized, controlled trial using low-dose CT.
  - Sponsored by the NCI and the American College of Radiology Imaging Network.
  - 7000 persons at high risk will be evaluated.
    - Participants will be assigned to either yearly low-dose CT (screening group) or no chest radiography (control group), in equal numbers.
    - The study was designed to detect a 50% reduction in cumulative mortality from lung cancer.

Imaging in lung cancer

Chest radiography

[Heitzman ER, *Semin Roentgenol* **12**: 165–174, 1977]
[Patz EG, *Chest* **117**: 90S–95S, 2000]
[Sider L, *Radiol Clin North Am* **28**: 583–597, 1990]
[Byrd RB, *Thorax* **24**: 573–575, 1969]
[Quinn D, *Chest* **110**: 1474–1479, 1996]

- Chest radiography remains the basic modality for the detection of lung cancer.
  [Quinn D, *Chest* **110**: 1474–1479, 1996]

- Lung cancer is more common in the right lung than in the left lung, and more common in the upper lobes, especially in the anterior segment.
  [Sider L, *Radiol Clin North Am* **28**: 583–597, 1990]

Central lesions

[Heitzman ER, *Semin Roentgenol* **12**: 165–174, 1977]

- Central lesions usually present as a combination of atelectasis, chronic obstructive pneumonia, and hilar mass.

- Atelectasis.
  - Common radiologic presentation in central tumors.
  - The endobronchial growth of the tumor may lead to bronchial obstruction and collapse of a segment, a lobe, or the entire lung.

19

- – If the lung collapse does not resolve following appropriate clinical management, the exclusion of endobronchial lesions becomes necessary.
- Chronic obstructive pneumonia.
  - – The pneumonia may be accompanied by some degree of collapse, but not infrequently appears as a uniform lobar or segmental opacificity without loss of volume.
- Hilar mass.
  - The growth of the malignant process through the bronchial wall and into the lung may result in a mass that is visible on radiographs.
  - Hilar adenopathy also may cause a convex bulge at the hila and may be asymmetric.
  - If the carcinoma has originated in a major bronchus, a hilar mass can be seen. However, when the growth has also occluded the bronchus, its extension into the lungs may be masked by the airless collapsed lung.
  - The mass in the collapsed segment may be identified because of its convex protrusion into adjacent aerated lung tissue.
  - The combination of a large central mass with partial collapse and post-obstructive pneumonia results in the typical radiographic sign called the 'S sign of Golden'.
  - The mass is composed of the convex bulging of the mass and a concave limb represented by the collapsed and elevated minor fissure caused by atelectasis.
    - – This is generally seen in right upper lobe collapse.
  - There is a tendency for central lung tumors to grow along the connective tissue sheath that encompasses the central bronchi and pulmonary arteries. These structures then become coated with the tumor.
    - – In the early stages of the disease, the mass adds little to the total bulk of the hilum.
  - The radiographic findings of mediastinal adenopathy include:
    - – wide mediastinum with lobulated contours
    - – thickening of the right paratracheal line
    - – convexity of the aortopulmonary window
    - – increase in the subcarinal density or convexity of the azygo-esophageal recess
    - – elevation of the hemidiaphragm from phrenic nerve involvement
    - – signs of superior vena cava syndrome.

- ↑ Density of the hilum when compared to the other side is usually a more reliable indicator of abnormality than absolute measurements of the hilar size.
- Central tumors may invade the lymphatic channels, producing lymphangitis carcinomatosa.
  - The lymphangitic spread of the tumor involving only one lobe or one lung is most likely the result of a primary lung cancer.
- Post contrast computerized tomography (CT) images are better at demonstrating the differential enhancement of atelectatic lung vs tumor mass.
  - The tumor mass is generally hypodense relative to the normal atelectatic lung.

Peripheral lesions

[Heitzman ER, *Semin Roentgenol* **12**: 165–174, 1977]

- Important features in the evaluation of a peripheral lesion are: size, border configuration, lobulation, corona radiata, peripheral line shadow, cavitation, calcification, and doubling time. These may help differentiate between benign and malignant nodules.

- Size.
  - In general, a mass > 4 cm in diameter will most often be diagnosed as a malignant tumor.
  - A lesion < 1 cm is generally <u>not</u> visible on chest radiography.
  - Malignant tumors may cross a fissure. This is very uncommon for inflammatory processes.

- Border.
  - Benign lesions are usually very sharply defined, whereas malignant lesions usually have ill-defined borders.

- Lobulation.
  - Caused by the tumor tissue advancing randomly into the adjacent lung.
  - Although it can also be seen in benign lesions, this finding favors a malignant process.

- Corona radiata.
  - Term used to describe fine and linear striations of the periphery of a mass.
  - Although it can be seen in silicosis and granulomas, this finding is highly suggestive of malignancy.

- Peripheral linear shadow.
  - Linear shadow extending from the lateral aspect of the peripheral lesions.
  - Although this can also be found in benign lesions, its presence favors a malignant process.

- Cavitation.
  - Relatively infrequent, occurring in about 2–4% of cases and, usually, as a late event.
  - The cavitated lesion is more likely to be malignant when the wall is thick or lobulated.

- Calcification.
  - Lesions that are diffusely or homogeneously calcified, those with stippled or ring-like calcification, and those with concentric calcification, are almost uniformly benign.
  - Calcifications are rarely seen in radiographs of lung cancer, although eccentric or amorphous calcifications have been reported in up to 6% of cases on CT images.
  - Sometimes, it represents the engulfment of a pre-existing granuloma.

- Doubling time.
  - As a general rule, if the lesion is unchanged in size after 2 years, it is most likely benign.
  - A doubling in size after 6 months to 2 years is more typical of adenocarcinoma.
  - A doubling time of < 6 months is usually indicative of an inflammatory process.

Squamous cell carcinoma

[Sider L, *Radiol Clin North Am* **28**: 583–597, 1990]
[Patz EG, *Chest* **117**: 90S–95S, 2000]

- Arises in the central bronchi in over 65% of cases.

- Initially, the tumor may be confined to the bronchial wall.
  - At this stage, it is clinically and radiographically silent.

- It frequently causes collapse and pneumonia, typically with absent air bronchograms.

- When the tumor invades the mediastinum, it is manifested on the chest radiograph as a lobulated widening of the mediastinum.

- When the tumor presents as a peripheral lesion, it is often very large.

- Squamous cell carcinoma is the cell type most frequently associated with cavitation, which results from central necrosis caused by ischemia.
  - Cavitation is present in 10–20% of cases, particularly in large peripheral lesions.
  - Cavities are usually thick and irregular; size range 0.5–3 cm.
  - Rarely, extensive necrosis may result in a thin-walled cavity.

- It is <u>the most common cause</u> of Pancoast tumor.

Adenocarcinomas

[Sider L, *Radiol Clin North Am* **28**: 583–597, 1990]
[Patz EG, *Chest* **117**: 90S–95S, 2000]

- Present as a peripheral mass in 60–70% of cases.

- The peripheral node is usually round or oval in shape.

- Hilar adenopathy is seen in 18% of cases and mediastinal adenopathy is seen in 2% of cases of peripheral adenocarcinoma.
  - Central lesions present with hilar adenopathy in 40% of cases and mediastinal adenopathy in 27% of cases.

- It may be associated with parenchymal scars and eccentric calcification.

- It may also present as a central mass without peripheral involvement, resembling squamous cell carcinoma.
  - The presentation of a peripheral nodule associated with a mediastinal or hilar mass is more common.

Bronchioloalveolar carcinoma

[Sider L, *Radiol Clin North Am* **28**: 583–597, 1990]
[Patz EG, *Chest* **117**: 90S–95S, 2000]

- Bronchioloalveolar carcinoma is a histologic subtype of adenocarcinoma that tends to grow along the pre-existing alveolar walls in a low-grade fashion.

- It usually presents as a solitary mass, an area of pneumonic infiltrate, or as multiple infiltrates.

- The most common presentation is a well-circumscribed nodule that remains unchanged in size over several years.

- A unique feature is the presence of air bronchograms.
- The CT angiogram sign.
  - Clearly visible vessels in a background of hazy ground glass opacity is now considered a too non-specific sign, as many benign processes also present similarly.

Large-cell carcinoma

[Sider L, *Radiol Clin North Am* **28**: 583–597, 1990]
[Patz EG, *Chest* **117**: 90S–95S, 2000]

- Presents as a peripheral mass in over 70% of cases.
- It is usually a rapidly growing mass.
  - The majority of the lesions are > 7 cm in diameter.
- The margins are poorly differentiated and lobulated.

Small-cell carcinoma

[Sider L, *Radiol Clin North Am* **28**: 583–597, 1990]

- The primary lesion is usually small and difficult to detect on radiographs.
- If it occurs endobronchially.
- The first sign is most typically a central mass that represents metastases to the ipsilateral hilar or mediastinal lymph nodes.
  - Hilar and mediastinal nodes are involved radiographically in 80% of cases at presentation, and in 100% of cases at autopsy.
  - The adenopathy is usually bulky in both the hilus and the mediastinum.

The changing radiographic presentation of lung cancer

- [Byrd RB, *Thorax* **24**: 573–575, 1969]
  In 1969, Byrd found that 62% of the adenocarcinomas and 31% of the squamous cell carcinomas presented with a peripheral lesion.
- [Quinn D, *Chest* **110**: 1474–1479, 1996]
  In 1996, Quinn found an increase in the incidence of adenocarcinomas presenting as a central lesion and squamous cell carcinomas presenting as a peripheral lesion.

- 46% of the adenocarcinomas were central (49% peripheral; 6% not classified).
- 43% of the squamous cell carcinomas were peripheral (51% central; 5% not classified).
- The other two cell types, small cell and large cell, did not have significant changes in location.

Computerized tomography

[Patz EF, *Radiology* **212**: 56–60, 1999]
[Hanson JA, *Eur Radiol* **7**: 161–172, 1997]
[Haberkorn U, *Lung Cancer* **34**: S13–S23, 2001]
[Webb RW, *Radiology* **178**: 705–713, 1991]

- Standard radiologic imaging modality used to stage lung cancer.

- Provides information about the primary lesion, thoracic lymph nodes, pleura, chest wall, and upper abdomen.

Lymph-node staging

[Hanson JA, *Eur Radiol* **7**: 161–172, 1997]

- Spread of tumor to hilar and mediastinal nodes is common at initial presentation of lung cancer, particularly with adenocarcinoma, central tumors, and tumors > 3 cm in size.

- The only substantial radiologic sign of nodal metastasis is enlargement.

- Adenopathy is defined by CT imaging as a lymph node > 1 cm in size in the short-axis diameter.
  - The use of node size to predict involvement by tumor has some limitations.
  - Normal subcarinal and lower paratracheal nodes may reach up to 15 mm in short-axis diameter, whereas those in the upper paratracheal region rarely exceed 7 mm, with hilar nodes generally being smaller than 3 mm.
  - Enlarged lymph nodes have many other causes, such as reactive hyperplasia to the primary tumor or distal infection, granulomatous infections, and inflammatory disorders.
    - Up to 2/3 of enlarged lymph nodes draining the post-obstructive pneumonia can be free from tumor.
    - Conversely, normal-sized lymph nodes may contain a microscopic tumor, a finding that appears to be a particular feature of adenocarcinoma.

- The Radiologic Diagnostic Oncologic Group (RDOG).
  [Webb RW, *Radiology* **178**: 705–713, 1991]
  - Found a sensitivity and specificity of 52% and 69%, respectively, for CT in the detection of mediastinal node metastases.
  - Magnetic resonance imaging (MRI) had a sensitivity and specificity of 48% and 64%, respectively.

Mediastinal and chest wall invasion

[Hanson JA, *Eur Radiol* **7**: 161–172, 1997]

- T_3 lesions are associated with invasion of the diaphragm, pericardium, mediastinal pleura, or chest wall, without involvement of the heart, great vessels, vertebral body, esophagus, or tracheal carina.

- Both CT and MRI can readily display extensive mediastinal disease.
  - However, both modalities are less accurate in determining lesser degrees of invasion.

- Chest wall invasion can only be diagnosed with confidence by CT if a large mass is seen or there is bone destruction.
  - These signs have a sensitivity of only 20%.

- The CT features may be used as a sign for successful surgical excision.
  (a) < 3 cm of mediastinal contact.
  (b) Maintained fat plane separating the tumor mass with mediastinum.
  (c) < 90% of circumferential aortic contact.
  - Mere contiguity does <u>not</u> imply infiltration, and an obtuse angle between the mass and the chest wall is an unreliable sign.
  - Pleural thickening, obliteration of the extrapleural fat plane, and extrapleural soft tissue can also be produced by reactive changes due to fibrosis and inflammation.

- The sensitivity and specificity of CT in differentiating T_{0-2} lesions from T_{3-4} lesions, according to RDOG, were 63% and 84%, respectively.
  - MRI in the same study had a sensitivity of 56% and a specificity of 80%.
    [Webb RW, *Radiology* **178**: 705–713, 1991]

Magnetic resonance imaging

[Htabu H, *Radiol Clin North Am* **38**: 593–620, 2000]
[Deslauriers J, *Chest* **117**: 96S–103S, 2000]

- As the lung produces little magnetic resonance signal, MRI is seldom used to evaluate the lung itself. However, the lungs produce a negative contrast, improving the visualization of the mediastinum.
  - Multiplanar and three-dimensional volume rendered images offer the surgeon a better perspective prior to excision.

- Although MRI has not been shown to be more accurate than CT in the evaluation of nodal disease and in the differentiation between T_{0-2} and T_{3-4} lesions, it may offer some advantages in certain situations due to its excellent delineation of the thoracic vessels.
  - MRI appears to be superior to CT in detecting mediastinal, chest wall tumor invasion into the heart and great vessels.
  - Pericardial invasion can be demonstrated very well, as the disruption of a low signal membrane.

- MRI is more accurate than CT in evaluating local invasion of superior sulcus tumors.
  - Particularly regarding their invasion into the vertebral body, spinal canal, brachial plexus, and subclavian artery.

- In patients with lung cancer who cannot tolerate iodinated contrast, MRI should be considered in addition to CT for the assessment of hilar and mediastinal involvement and lymph node metastases.

- Dynamic, cine MRI during breathing can demonstrate lack of adherence of a tumor to the adjacent chest wall.
  - However, it cannot differentiate between benign and malignant processes.

Positron emission tomography

[Czernin J, *Annu Rev Med* **53**: 89–112, 2002]
[Lowe VJ, *Thorax* **53**: 703–712, 1998]
[Pieterman RM, *N Engl J Med* **343**: 254–261, 2000]
[Laking G, *Thorax* **56**(Suppl II): 38–44, 2001]
[Kalff V, *J Clin Oncol* **19**: 111–118, 2001]

Background

- Whole-body positron emission tomography (PET) imaging is a molecular imaging modality that detects metabolic changes in tumor cells.

- The most commonly used tracer is the [^{18}F]deoxyglucose (FDG).

- Tumor cells rely on adenosine 5'-triphosphate (ATP) generated from glycolysis to meet the energy requirements of rapidly replicating tissue.
  - With the loss of efficient production of ATP by the Krebs cycle in the transformed neoplastic cells, there is an associated 19-fold increase in glucose consumption per mole of ATP produced.
- After intravenous injection, FDG is taken up by tumor cells and phosphorylated by hexokinase to FDG-6-phosphate.
  - Unlike glucose 6-phosphate, FDG-6-phosphate is not metabolized in the glycolytic pathway and remains trapped intracellularly, providing a record of glycolysis in cells throughout the body, which is scanned 45–60 minutes after the injection of FDG.
- PET imaging provides numerical data by quantitating the number of positron emissions.
  - These data accurately reflect the amount of FDG accumulating in a selected region.
  - The standardized uptake ratio (SUR) is a value of the uptake normalized for the patient's body weight and imaging dose.
  - SUR values > 2.5 have been considered indicative of malignancy.
- Possible causes of false-positive FDG-PET include: infection, acute inflammation, recent surgical wound, and muscle hypermetabolism.
- Possible causes of false-negative FDG-PET include: low-grade malignancy, microscopic or small focal malignancy, hyperglycemia, and adjacent highly metabolic focus.
  - The main contraindication for PET is hyperglycemia, which interferes with tissue uptake and causes false-negative results.
  - Bronchioloalveolar and carcinoid tumors have demonstrated low FDG accumulation in some series.
  - Occasionally, well differentiated adenocarcinomas may have a relatively less marked increase in FDG accumulation, although the SUR is still abnormal.
  - All other types of primary lung cancer, regardless of degree of differentiation, present with increased FDG accumulation.
  - FDG may accumulate as part of the physiologic processes in the brain and urinary tract, making the evaluation of metastases at these sites difficult.
- The potential disadvantage of PET is the limited anatomical resolution.
  - Which may make unreliable the evaluation of the extent of primary tumor, especially if there is mediastinal invasion.

Role of PET in the diagnosis and staging of lung cancer

- PET improves the rate of detection of local and distant metastases in patients with non-small-cell cancer.

- When compared to traditional staging methods, PET can result in a more accurate classification of the stage of disease in patients with resectable, non-small-cell lung cancer.
  - A PET scan is the most accurate non-invasive method available for characterizing mediastinal node status in the preoperative staging of non-small-cell lung cancer.
  - PET is also equally reliable and accurate for detecting disease in small and large lymph node lesions, with better efficacy than CT. [Gupta NC, *Chest* **117**: 773–778, 2000]
  - Farrel suggests that in patients with stage I, non-small-cell lung cancer a negative PET scan indicates that mediastinoscopy is unnecessary and patients can proceed directly to thoracotomy. [Farrel MA, *Radiology* **215**: 886–890, 2000]

- Eight studies from 1994 to 1997 compared PET and CT in the mediastinal staging of lung cancer.
  - 339 patients were evaluated.
  - Sensitivity of PET was 88% (range 75–100%) and specificity was 93% (range 81–100%).
  - Sensitivity of CT was 63% (range 43–81%) and specificity was 80% (range 44–94%).
  - The difference was statistically significant in 7/8 studies.

- Pieterman reported a sensitivity and specificity of PET for the detection of mediastinal metastases of 91% and 86%, respectively.
  - The corresponding values for CT were 75% and 66%, respectively.
  - The combination of PET and CT did not significantly improve the sensitivity and specificity, which were 94% and 86%, respectively.
  - Overall, compared with CT, the use of PET indicated a different stage of the cancer in 62 of the 102 patients evaluated. The stage was raised in 42 patients and lowered in 20 patients.

- PET detects not only unsuspected metastases, but also many false-positive findings on CT scan can be correctly interpreted as negative, allowing patients with otherwise unresectable tumors to be surgical candidates.
  - Three studies done from 1994 to 1996 evaluated the detection of unsuspected metastases with PET.
  - 194 patients were evaluated in the three studies combined.

- At least 10% of patients were found to have distant metastases not otherwise detected by routine chest CT scans.
- Kalff evaluated the clinical impact of FDG-PET in patients with non-small-cell lung cancer.
  - 105 patients were evaluated.
  - 70 patients showed a change or influence of the therapy.
  - Aggressive therapy was prevented in 27 of 78 (35%) patients initially planned for treatment with curative intent by identifying more advanced disease than was previously suspected.
  - PET also allowed 4 of 16 (25%) patients initially considered for palliative therapy to be offered potentially curative treatment.

Conclusions

- The addition of PET to comprehensive conventional evaluation of non-small-cell lung cancer can have a significant impact on clinical management.

- More accurate staging can spare a substantial number of patients the morbidity related to futile attempts to aggressively control the disease.

- PET staging can also provide a chance of survival in a small but significant number of patients who would have been denied potentially curative therapy based on false-positive structural imaging studies.

- PET-CT hybrids are superior to CT scans, PET scans, or the visual correlation of PET scans plus CT scans.

- [Lardinois D, N Engl J Med **348**: 2500–2507, 2003]
  A Swiss study of 50 patients, comparing the accuracy of tumor staging using PET-CT, CT scan alone, PET scan alone, or visual correlation by a radiologist of the CT scan and PET scan.
  - RESULTS:
    - Better tumor staging with PET-CT.
    - CT alone ($p = 0.001$).
    - PET alone ($p < 0.001$).
    - Visual correlation of CT + PET ($p = 0.013$).

- PET scans may be very helpful, predicting tumor response much sooner than CT scans.
  [Weber WA, J Clin Oncol **21**: 2651–2657, 2003]
  - Response Assessment Study.
    - 57 patients with stage IIIB or IV non-small-cell lung cancer.

- FDG-PET was done before and after 21 days of first cycle of platinum-based chemotherapy.
- 28 responders, 27 non-responders.
- Close correlation between metabolic response and best response according to Response Evaluation Criteria Solid Tumors (RECIST) criteria.
- RESULTS:
  - Median time to progression → 163 days vs 54 days.
  - Median survival → 252 days vs 151 days.

5

Diagnostic techniques in lung cancer

This chapter and the imaging chapter (Chapter 4) are devoted to lung cancer diagnosis.

[Schreiber G, *Chest* **123**(Suppl): 115s–128s, 2003]
[Rivera P, *Chest* **123**(Suppl): 129s–136s, 2003]
[Toloza EM, *Chest* **123**(Suppl): 157s–166s, 2003]

Introduction

- Clinical and radiological findings should guide the diagnostic approach, depending on the size and location of the tumor, the presence of metastatic disease, and the clinical status of the patient.

- Diagnostic and staging work-up is often undertaken concomitantly.

- Clinical judgment is important in maximizing sensitivity while avoiding unnecessary procedures.

- Priority should be given to the procedure that provides both a diagnosis and the highest stage of the tumor.
  - Fine needle aspiration (FNA) of liver metastasis or pleural effusion in patient with radiographic evidence of lung tumor.

General approach

- In suspected small-cell lung cancer the easiest method should be applied according to the clinical presentation (sputum cytology, thoracentesis, FNA, bronchoscopy with/without transbronchial needle aspiration (TBNA), transthoracic needle aspiration (TTNA)).

- In patients with pleural effusion, thoracentesis should be attempted first, followed by repeat thoracentesis, and then thoracoscopy if the cytology is inconclusive.

- Patients with a solitary extrapulmonary metastasis should have the distant site assessed by FNA as a first step.

- When biopsy of the distant site is unsafe, biopsy of the primary lung lesion should be attempted by the safest possible method (e.g. sputum cytology, thoracentesis, FNA, bronchoscopy), as clinically indicated.

- In patients with no evidence of distal involvement but with suspected mediastinal nodes, the latter site should be assessed.

- When a solitary peripheral nodule is suggestive of cancer, excisional biopsy, followed by anatomic lung resection if the diagnosis is confirmed, is the preferred approach.

Sputum cytology

- Accuracy depends on sampling, preservation techniques, tumor location, and the cytopathologist's experience.

- At least three specimens should be submitted.

- The average sensitivity and specificity in a compilation of 16 studies were 66% and 99%, respectively.

- In one report the sensitivity for central lesions was 71% vs 49% for peripheral lesions.

- A 3-day collection of early morning sputum, preserved in Saccomano's solution, appears to be the optimum method of assessment.

Flexible bronchoscopy

- The least invasive method.

- In endobronchial disease the sensitivity of endobronchial biopsies was 74%; with brushings alone it was 59%, and with washings alone it was 48%.

- The overall sensitivity for all modalities was 88% in one review (3,754 patients).
- The addition of transbronchoscopic needle aspirate (TBNA) ↑ the sensitivity (76%) and specificity (96%), but the negative predictive value is only (71%).
- The sensitivity of bronchoscopy for peripheral lesions depends on:
  - The size of the lesion, the use of fluoroscopy and TBNA: one study reported a sensitivity of 62% vs 33% in patients with peripheral tumors sized > 2 cm or < 2 cm, respectively.
- Recently introduced:
  - Endobronchial, ultrasound-guided, needle aspirate (EBUS) of mediastinal lesions; bronchoscopy with electromagnetic navigation-guided transbronchial lung biopsies of peripheral nodules.

Transthoracic needle aspiration

- In a review representing 11,279 patients, an overall sensitivity of 97% and a specificity of 99% were reported.
- The sensitivity for lesions > 2 cm or < 2 cm in size was not statistically significant.
- CT guidance has a higher sensitivity than fluoroscopic guidance.
- For peripheral lung lesions the sensitivity of TTNA is greater than that of bronchoscopy.
- False-negative rates are in the range 20–30%.
  - Making this an unreliable method for ruling out suspicious solitary lesions, which should be approached by excisional biopsy.

Mediastinoscopy and mediastinostomy

- One review of 5,687 patients in 14 studies detected an overall sensitivity of 81%, with a negative predictive value of 91% for mediastinoscopy.
- Anterior mediastinostomy (Chamberlain procedure) can be used to assess lymph-node stations 2R, 3, and 4R when performed through the right side, and stations 5 and 6 when performed through the left side.
  - This procedure has a sensitivity of 60–80%.

Accuracy in differentiating non-small-cell and small-cell lung cancers

- In a review of 21 studies with 6,305 patients:
  - Of patients initially diagnosed as having non-small-cell lung cancer (NSCLC), 2% actually had small-cell lung cancer (SCLC), and 9% of patients initially diagnosed as having SCLC actually had NSCLC.

- If the clinical presentation is not usual for the pathologic diagnosis, a second biopsy should be contemplated.

Esophageal, endoscopic, ultrasound-guided, fine needle aspiration

[Gress FG, *Ann Intern Med* **127**(8 Pt 1): 604–612, 1997]
[LeBlanc JK, *Chest* **123**(5): 1718–1725, 2003]

- A pooled analysis of five studies (215 patients) using esophageal, endoscopic, ultrasound-guided, fine needle aspiration (EUS FNA) in the diagnosis of mediastinal involvement showed an overall sensitivity of 88%, with a specificity of 91% and a negative predictive value of 77%.
  - EUS FNA is superior to CT in the mediastinal staging of lung cancer.

- EUS guided biopsy of the mediastinal nodes can be performed with high accuracy in mediastinal American Thoracic Society stations 5, 7, 8, and 9.
  - Most left paratracheal nodes can also be biopsied through the esophagus.
  - Pretracheal nodes are not sampled using EUS FNA.
  - Lung tumors situated in posterior segments adjacent to the esophagus can also be safely biopsied using EUS FNA.

- EUS trucut biopsy (EUS TCB) may ↑ the accuracy of EUS-guided tissue sampling when combined with FNA.

- EUS also allows visualization of lesions in the left lobe of the liver, left adrenal gland, or celiac nodes, all of which are sites of potential metastasis in lung cancer.

- EUS FNA allows tissue acquisition from lymph nodes < 10 mm, which is beyond the resolution of a CT scan.

- EUS FNA combined with PET provides > 90% sensitivity in the mediastinal staging of NSCLC.

Lung pathology

[Rosai J, *Ackerman's Surgical Pathology*, 9th edn. Philadelphia, PA, Mosby-Year Book, 1996]

[Sternberg S, *Diagnostic Surgical Pathology*, 3rd edn. Philadelphia, PA, Lippincott Williams & Wilkins, 1999]

[Travis W, *World Health Organization Classification of Tumors: Tumors of the Lung, Pleura, Thymus, and Heart*. Lyon, IARC Press, 2004]

Carcinoma

Epidemiology

- The number 1 cause of cancer death in the USA, ♂ and ♀.

- Peak ages: 50–69 years.

- 2% occur before age 40 years.

- Cigarette smoking causes most cases of lung cancer.

- Rare in Asians.

Etiology

- Cigarette smoking causes most cases.

- Radiation exposure: uranium and radon.

- Asbestos, nickel, chromate, coal, mustard gas.

- Arsenic, beryllium, iron, vinyl chloride, gold mining.

Symptoms

- Cough.
- Weight loss.
- Chest pain.
- Shortness of breath.
- ↑ sputum.

Systemic symptoms

- Lambert–Eaton myasthenic syndrome.
- Sensory peripheral neuropathy.
- Acanthosis nigricans.
- Leukomoid reaction.
- Hypertrophic pulmonary osteoarthropathy.
- Superior vena cava syndrome.
- Ulnar nerve and Horner's syndrome (Pancoast tumors).

Classification

- Non-small-cell carcinoma (NSCLC) (80%).
- Small-cell carcinoma (SCLC) (20%).
- 50% NSCLCs are metastatic at diagnosis vs 80% of SCLCs.
- Many have mixed histologic subtypes.

Spread

- Along bronchus, into lung parenchyma, to mediastinum or pleura.
- Cause pleural seeding, pleural effusion.
- Diaphragm and chest wall involvement.

Metastasis

- 50% have nodal involvement at resection.
  - Hilar, mediastinal, and supraclavicular.

- Adrenal glands (50%), liver (30%), brain, and bone.
- Opposite lung, pericardium, and kidneys.

Treatment

- Excision (NSCLC).
- Radiation therapy (usually non-curative).
- Chemotherapy (rarely curative, even for SCLC).

Survival

- 10–15% → 5-year survival.
- 30% have limited disease at diagnosis (resection for cure an option).
- Stage I NSCLC, 5-year survival → 60%.

Poor prognostic factors

- High TNM stage.
- Weight loss > 10%.
- Age < 40 years.
- ♀ (usually are high stage).
- Pleural effusion.
- Tumor size > 3 cm.
- Lack of lymphoplasmacytic reaction.
- Small cell/giant cell subtypes.
- Lymphovascular invasion (LVI).
- p53 (+), HER2 (+).
  [Han H, *Hum Pathol* **22**: 105–110, 2002]

Favorable subtypes

- Non-mucinous bronchioloalveolar carcinoma.
- Well-differentiated, squamous cell carcinoma (SCC).

Gross

- Central tumors: SCC and small-cell carcinoma.
- Peripheral tumors: usually adenocarcinomas.

Microscopy

- Begins with atypia, then warty excrescence, then fungates into lumen, and penetrates the wall of the bronchus, growing along a broad front to produce a cauliflower-like intraparenchymal mass.
  - 80% have vascular invasion.

Molecular

- EGFR (+) in 84% of SCCs.
- *HER2/neu* (+) and *K-ras* (+) frequent in adenocarcinoma; infrequent in SCC.
- p53 mutations frequent in all types of lung cancer.
- C-myc (small-cell carcinomas).
- Disruption of Rb gene is universal in lung cancer.
- Allelic losses of 3p is present in both SCC and adenocarcinoma.
- Loss of Cables protein expression (NSCLC) at 18q11-12. [Tan D, *Hum Pathol* **34**: 143–149, 2003]

Squamous cell carcinoma

[Ogino S, *Hum Pathol* **33**: 1052–1054, 2002]
[Wang BY, *Hum Pathol* **33**: 921–926, 2002]

- Usually ♂ and smokers.
- Most common type of lung cancer in western countries.
- May cause hypercalcemia due to production of parathyroid-hormone-related protein.
- Central cases arise from bronchial epithelial dysplasia.
- Peripheral cases usually lack dysplasia.
- Symptoms: bronchial obstruction.

- Cytology: often (+) in sputum.
- Gross:
  - Central portion of lung affects larger bronchi.
  - May be peripheral.
  - Invades peribronchial soft tissue, lung parenchyma, and nearby nodes.
  - May compress pulmonary artery and vein.
  - Peripheral tumors are often nodular, with central necrosis/ cavitation.
  - Surrounding lung has lipid pneumonia, bronchopneumonia, atelectasis.
  - Calcification is unusual.
- Microscopy:
  - Sheets/islands of large polygonal malignant cells containing keratin.
  - Adjacent bronchial dysplasia or carcinoma in situ is common.
  - May have focal areas of intracytoplasmic mucin.
  - May have clear cell change (glycogen).
  - Variants: small, clear, papillary, basaloid, spindle cell.
    - Basaloid: very aggressive clinical course.
  - Positive stains:
    - High molecular weight keratin (HMWK; 34BE12), keratin 5/6, epithelial membrane antigen (EMA), S100 protein, CD15, carcinoembryonic antigen (CEA), p53, p63, human papilloma virus (HPV).
  - Negative stains:
    - vimentin, TTF-1, Ck7.
  - Differential diagnosis:
    - Squamous metaplasia with atypia in diffuse alveolar damage.
    - Thymic SCC.
    - Large-cell carcinoma.

Small-cell carcinoma

[Rossi G, *Mod Pathol* **16**: 1041–1047, 2003]
[Nicholson SA, *Am J Surg Pathol* **26**: 1184–1197, 2002]
[Matsuki Y, *Mod Pathol* **16**: 72–78, 2003]

- Also called undifferentiated or oat-cell carcinoma.
- Account for 10–20% of all lung carcinomas.
- Usually ♂ and smokers.
- Median age → 60 years.
- Very aggressive, with early mediastinal node involvement.

- Derived from primitive cells of basal bronchial epithelium.

- Associated with paraneoplastic syndromes including:
  - Syndromes associated with production of ADH, ACTH, parathyroid hormone, calcitonin, gonadotropins, and serotonin.
  - Encephalomyelitis.
  - Sensory neuropathy.
  - Lambert–Eaton syndrome.

- Biopsies often crushed.

- Flow cytometry: CD56 (+), CD45 (–).
  [Cornfield D, *Arch Pathol Lab Med* **127**: 461–464, 2003]

- Treatment: chemotherapy, radiation.

- Cure rates → 15–25% for limited disease.

- Most have extended disease and live ~ 1 year.

- Gross:
  - Usually central/hilar.
  - White-tan.
  - Soft.
  - Friable.
  - Extensive necrosis.
  - Peripheral nodules with well-defined border.
  - Fleshy cut surface.

- Microscopy:
  - Small to medium sized round/oval cells.
  - Hyperchromatic.
  - Minimal cytoplasm with nuclear molding.
  - Salt and pepper chromatin.
    - Cells in sheets, ribbons, clusters, rosettes, or peripheral pallisading.
  - Azzopardi phenomenon:
    - No glands.
    - Common necrosis and apoptotic debris.
    - May have larger cells with similar morphology.
    - May have small mixtures of SCC or adenocarcinoma.
    - Rarely, scattered giant cells.

- Positive stains:
  - Pan-keratin (dot like pattern), TTF-1, histamine decarboxylase, CD117, chromogranin, synaptophysin, CD56.

- Negative stains:
  - CD45, CD99, p63.

- Differential diagnosis:
  - Carcinoids (all types): less necrosis, mitosis, apoptosis than SCC.
  - Small, blue, round cell tumors, for example: peripheral neuroecto-dermal tumor, CD99 (+), keratin (–), TTF-1 (–).
  - Poorly differentiated non-small cell carcinoma.
  - Lymphoma CD45 (+), keratin (–).
  - Lymphocytes of inflammation.
  - Merkel carcinoma: CK20 (+), CK7 (–), TTF-1 (–).

Adenocarcinoma

[Terracciano LM, Am J Surg Pathol **27**: 1302–1312, 2003]
[Miettinen M, Am J Surg Pathol **27**: 150–158, 2003]
[Yatabe Y, Am J Surg Pathol **26**: 767–773, 2002]
[Terasaki H, Am J Surg Pathol **27**: 937–951, 2003]

- Arises from terminal bronchioles.

- In the USA accounts for 50% of lung carcinomas in ♀.

- Most common subtype in non-smokers.

- 80% contain mucin.

- Grows slower than SCCs.

- May be associated with scarring.

- 5-year survival: stage I, 69%; stage II, 40%; stage IIIA, 17%; stage IIIB, 5%; stage IV, 8%.

- Peripheral tumors with bronchioloalveolar and invasive areas < 5 mm had low rates of vascular/pleural invasion and no nodal involvement.

- More likely TTF-1 (–) in ♂ or smokers.

- Gross: 77% involve visceral pleura, producing puckering/pleural retraction.

- 65% are peripheral.

- Usually not cavitary.

- Often associated with a peripheral scar or honeycombing.

- Rarely spreads into the pleural space to coat visceral/parietal pleura.

- Major histologic subtypes:
  - Bronchoalveolar.
  - Acinar adenocarcinoma.
  - Papillary adenocarcinoma.
  - Solid with mucin production.

- Cellular differentiation within subtypes:
  - Bronchial surface cell type with little/no mucin.
  - Goblet cell type.
  - Bronchial gland cell type.
  - Clara cell type (50%).
  - Type II alveolar epithelial cell type.
  - Hepatoid: aggressive.

- Tumors $\leq$ 1.5 cm are usually one cell type.
  - Larger tumors are often mixed.

- Vascular invasion common.

- Rarely, choriocarcinoma foci, pagetoid spread along bronchial mucosa, eosinophilic intracytoplasmic globules, clear cell change (glycogen).

- Periphery of tumor often has minimal atypia, with marked atypia centrally.

- Positive stains:
  - Mucin, LMWK (CK7), EMA, CEA, TTF-1 (72%), surfactant apoprotein (50%), p53.

- Negative stains:
  - CK20, vimentin, keratin 5, P504S.

- Differential diagnosis:
  - Metastatic adenocarcinoma: multiple lesions, morphological homogeneous.
  - Epitheliod mesothelioma.
  - Reactive pneumocyte atypical (scars, organizing alveolar injury).

Subtypes of adenocarcinoma

Bronchioloalveolar carcinoma

[Lau SK, *Mod Pathol* **15**: 538–542, 2002]
[Shah RN, *Hum Pathol* **33**: 915–920, 2002]

- Arises from alveolar walls.

- 1–9% of all lung carcinomas; ♂ = ♀.
- Solitary lesions can be resected (5-year survival ~ 50%).
- Overall 5-year survival ~ 25%.
- Late metastasis.
- More favorable prognosis:
  - Non-mucinous histology (hobnail cells, Clara cells).
  - Localized disease.
- Has lepidic spread (along alveolar septa).
- If stromal/vascular/pleural invasion seen, designated adenocarcinoma, mixed.
- Gross: in lung periphery, nodule(s), or pneumonia-like infiltrate.
- Microscopy:
  - Tall columnar cells line up along alveolar septa.
  - Cells project into spaces with papillary projections.
  - Underlying lung architecture preserved.
  - Usually well differentiated.
  - Mucinous (Clara or type II alveolar epithelial cells).
  - Non-mucinous types (goblet cells).
  - May have PAS (+) intranuclear inclusions.
- Positive stains:
  - α-1-Antitrypsin (Clara cells), surfactant (type 2 pneumocytes), TTF-1 (most non-mucinous), CK7.
- Negative stains:
  - CK20 (but 25–90% of mucinous are CK20 (+)).
- Differential diagnosis:
  - Metastatic mucinous carcinoma.

Papillary adenocarcinoma

- Papillary structures with true fibrovascular core should comprise at least 75% of tumor.
- Necrosis and lung invasion may be present.

Micropapillary adenocarcinoma

[Miyoshi T, *Am J Surg Pathol* **27**: 101–109, 2003]
[Amin MB, *Am J Surg Pathol* **26**: 358–364, 2002]

- Associated with nodal/intrapulmonary metastasis.
- Seen in non-smokers.
- Poorer survival than non-papillary for stage I.
- Microscopy:
  - Small papillary tufts without a fibrovascular core.
  - Associated with varied other histologic subtypes.
- Positive stains:
  - CK7, TTF-1.

Acinar adenocarcinoma

- Composed of acini or tubules.
- Has columnar or cuboidal cells, which may be mucin producing.
- Resemble bronchial gland or bronchial lining epithelial cells.

Other subtypes

- Fetal adenocarcinoma.
- Mucinous cystadenocarcinoma.
- Signet-ring-cell adenocarcinoma.
- Clear-cell adenocarcinoma.

- Fetal adenocarcinoma.
  - Mean age of presentation ~ 40 years.
  - Better prognosis than pulmonary blastoma.
  - Variant of bronchioloalveolar carcinoma.
  - Associated with upregulation of Wnt signaling pathway.
  - Gross: well-defined, no capsule, not related to bronchi.
  - Microscopy:
    - Irregular tubular structures of columnar epithelial cells.
    - Clear cytoplasm and oval nuclei, continuous with morules.
    - Fibrous stroma without atypia.
  - Positive stains:
    - chromogranin A, synaptophysin, N-CAM.
  - Negative stains:
    - p53.
- Mucinous 'colloid' adenocarcinoma.
  - Identical to counterpart in gastrointestinal tract.
  - Dissecting mucin pools with neoplastic epithelial islands.

- Mucinous cystadenocarcinoma.
  - Circumscribed.
  - Partial fibrous tissue capsule.
  - Central cystic changes with mucin pooling.
  - Neoplastic mucinous epithelium growth along alveolar walls.
- Signet ring cell adenocarcinoma.
  - Usually focal pattern associated with other histologic subtypes.
  - Exclusion of metastasis from gastrointestinal tract is necessary.
  - Aggressive.
- Clear cell adenocarcinoma.
  - Mostly a focal morphological feature.
  - Is rarely a major component of a tumor.
  - Metastatic renal cell carcinoma is a major consideration.

Large cell undifferentiated carcinoma

- May be undifferentiated SCC or adenocarcinoma.
- Diagnosis of exclusion.
- 80% of patients ♂.
- Associated with eosinophilia and leukocytosis (tumor production of cerebrospinal fluid).
- Behavior is similar to adenocarcinoma.
- 5-year survival:
  - Stage I, 65%; stage II, 26%; stage IIIA, 18%; stage IIIB, 15%; stage IV, 6%.
- Gross:
  - Usually peripheral lung.
  - Spherical tumor with well-defined borders.
  - Bulging, fleshy, homogenous gray-white cut surface.
  - No anthracosis.
  - Frequently involves thoracic wall.
- Microscopy:
  - Large polygonal/anaplastic cells.
  - Solid nest growth.
  - No squamous/glandular differentiation.
  - Vesicular nuclei.
  - Prominent nucleoli.

- Moderately abundant cytoplasm.
- Well-defined cell borders.

- Positive stains:
  - Keratin 5 (56%); calretinin (38%); thrombomodulin (25%); mesothelin (13%); TTF-1 (variable).

Large-cell neuroendocrine carcinoma

- Resembles a non-small-cell carcinoma.

- May have subtle neuroendocrine architecture confirmed by special stains.

- Microscopy:
  - Larger tumor cells than atypical carcinoid.
  - High nuclear grade.
  - Prominent nucleoli.
  - ↑ mitotic activity.
  - Necrosis
  - Variable neuroendocrine architecture (pallisading /rosettes).

- Positive stains:
  - Synaptophysin, CD117 (60%), F1 (50%), chromogranin.

Lymphoepithelioma-like carcinoma

[Xhabg YL, *Am J Surg Pathol* **26**: 715–723, 2002]

- Rare.

- More frequent in China.

- Most patients → ♀, non-smokers.

- Rare in Caucasians, and usually Epstein–Barr virus (EBV) (–).

- Tumor size may correlate with EBV serology titer.

- May have better prognosis than other NSCLC of lung.

- Gross:
  - Well-circumscribed nodules.

- Microscopy:
  - Syncytial growth of epithelial cells.
  - Large vesicular nuclei.
  - Prominent eosinophilic nucleoli.

- Accompanied by marked CD8 (+) lymphocytic infiltration.
- Predominantly pushing borders.
- Permeative interface with adjacent lung.
- Occasional amyloid deposition.

• Positive stains:
  - EBV, EBER-1, LMP, bcl2, patchy keratin.

• Negative stains:
  - CD45.

• Differential diagnosis:
  - Metastatic nasopharyngeal carcinoma.
  - Lymphoma.
  - Inflammatory pseudotumor.

Adenosquamous carcinoma

• Substantial amounts of squamous and glandular differentiation.

• < 10% of lung carcinomas.

• 90% peripheral, often associated with scars.

• Metastasis may have different histology.

• Poorer prognosis than either component alone.

• Positive stains:
  - AE1/AE3, CAM5.2, CK7, EMA, TTF-1 (adenoma component).

• Negative stains:
  - Usually CK20.

• Differential diagnosis:
  - Entrapped alveolar/bronchiolar acini within SCC.
  - Adenoma associated with squamous metaplasia.
  - Mucoepidermoid carcinoma.

Sarcomatoid carcinoma

[Pelosi G, *Am J Surg Pathol* **27**: 1203–1215, 2003]
[Rossi G, *Am J Surg Pathol* **27**: 311–324, 2003]

• Also called pleomorphic, spindle cell, giant-cell carcinoma, pulmonary blastoma, carcinosarcoma.

• < 1% of all carcinomas.

- Mean age → 65 years.
- Mostly ♂ and smokers.
- Presumed epithelial origin.
- Epithelial and sarcomatous components express common markers differently.
- Common nodal metastasis.
- Stage I tumors have same prognosis as other stage I NSCLCs.
- Higher stage tumors have worse prognosis by stage than other NSCLCs.
- Metastasize to same areas as NSCLCs.
- Metastasize to unusual sites: small intestine, rectum, kidney, esophagus.

Carcinosarcoma

[Dacic S, *Am J Surg Pathol* **26**: 510–516, 2002]

- Carcinoma component is combined with a sarcoma.
- Sarcoma consists of heterologous elements: malignant cartilage/bone/muscle.
- The two components appear to have a common origin.
- Gross:
  - 2–17 cm.
  - Necrosis.
  - Hemorrhage.
- Microscopy:
  - NSCLC with at least 10% neoplastic spindle/giant cells.
  - Usually with epithelial cells.
  - Epithelial component 10–85%.
  - Adenocarcinoma, large-cell carcinoma, SCC.
  - Spindle cells: resemble malignant peripheral nerve sheath tumor, malignant fibrous histiocytoma, or fibrosarcoma.
  - Bizarre giant cells with multilobulated nuclei.
  - Stroma often myxoid.
  - Frequent inflammatory infiltrate.
  - Collagen fibers.
  - Numerous mitoses.
  - Common necrosis and vascular invasion.

- Positive stains:
  - Cytokeratin, K7, TTF, vimentin, smooth muscle markers.
- Negative stains:
  - CK20.
- Molecular:
  - Allelic loss in carcinosarcomas at 3p, 5q, 17p.

Giant cell carcinoma

- Carcinomas with pleomorphic, sarcomatoid, or sarcomatous elements.
- < 1% of all primary lung carcinomas.
- Microscopy:
  - Highly pleomorphic giant cells.
  - Often in inflammatory stroma with emperipolesis.
  - Giant cells are multinucleated (syncytiotrophoblast like).
- Positive stains:
  - TTF-1 may be positive.
- Negative stains:
  - Surfactant apoprotein A.
- Differential diagnosis:
  - Primary and metastatic sarcomas.
    1. Pleomorphic rhabdomyosarcoma.
    2. Metastatic adrenocortical.
    3. Metastatic choriocarcinoma.
       - Focal β-HCG seen in NSCLC; do not call these chorio-carcinoma.
  - Teratoma.

Pulmonary blastoma

- Also called embryoma.
- Considered a subtype of pleomorphic carcinoma/carcinosarcoma.
- Usually adults.
- 20% of patients < 20 years old.
- Metastasis common.
- 2/3 die within 2 years.

- In infants/children, epithelial component is benign appearing or minimal.
- Stroma may be rhabdomyoblastic or chondroid.
- Tumors may be cystic and may involve pleura and lung.
- Gross:
  - Peripheral.
  - Solitary.
  - Well circumscribed.
  - Large.
- Microscopy:
  - Biphasic tumor.
  - Epithelial/mesenchymal components look primitive/'fetal type'.
  - Well-formed, tubular glands surrounded by cellular stroma.
- Glandular cells:
  - Tall.
  - Columnar.
  - Clear cytoplasm.
  - Subnuclear/supranuclear cytoplasmic vacuoles.
- Morules with ground-glass nuclei are common.
- Stroma may differentiate to:
  - Striated muscle.
  - Smooth muscle.
  - Cartilage.
- Positive stains:
  - Adenocarcinoma component: keratin, EMA, CEA, chromogranin (+/−), calcitonin (+/−), gastrin-releasing peptide (+/−), bombesin (+/−), somatostatin (+/−), serotonin (+/−).
  - Stromal component: vimentin, muscle-specific actin, desmin (if striated muscle present), S100 (if cartilage present), keratin (−/+).

Dysplasia/carcinoma in situ

- Associated with bronchial lesions.
- Seen in normal bronchus near carcinoma.
- Gross: normal, papillary, or granular mucosa.
- Microscopy − squamous cells replace respiratory-type epithelium:
  - Focally to full thickness.

- ↑ nuclear/cytoplasmic ratio.
- Nuclear pleomorphism.
- Mitotic activity.
- Intact basement membrane with no invasion.
- Submucosal gland ducts may be involved.

Bronchoalveolar atypical adenomatous hyperplasia

[Nakanishi K, *Hum Pathol* **33**: 697–702, 2002]

- Continuum from adenoma to well-differentiated bronchoalveolar carcinoma.
- Diagnostic variability exists
- Associated with bronchoalveolar and papillary adenocarcinoma.
- Gross: seen as a focal lesion.
- Low-grade and high-grade lesions with progressive ↑ telomerase.
- Microscopy:
  - Cuboidal cells replace alveolar lining cells:
    - Uniform, mildly to highly atypical nuclei.
    - Minimal mitotic figures.

Carcinoid and related tumors

Carcinoid tumor

- Also called well-differentiated neuroendocrine carcinoma.
- < 5% of primary lung tumors.
- Locally invasive, rarely metastasizes.
- Usually ≤ 40 years of age.
- No gender predilection.
- Not related to smoking.
- Occasionally occurs as part of multiple endocrine neoplasia (MEN) syndrome.
- May infiltrate or spread to local lymph nodes, not affecting prognosis.
- Rarely, causes carcinoid syndrome.
- 10-year survival → 50%.

- Gross:
  - Either central (polypoid and endobronchial in major bronchi) or peripheral (solid/nodular).
  - Usually well defined.
  - Smooth, ivory to pink, cut surface.
  - No necrosis.

- Microscopy:
  - Nests or trabeculae of medium sized polygonal cells.
  - Low nuclear grade.
  - Round to oval, finely granular nuclei.
  - Lightly eosinophilic cytoplasm.
  - May have rosettes or small acinar structures.
  - Variable mucin.
  - Scanty vascular stroma.
  - Occasionally amyloid stroma with bone.
  - No or minimal mitotic activity or necrosis.

Central carcinoid tumor

- Most common type.

- Slow growing.

- Associated with obstruction, infection, hemorrhage.

- Usually adults, but also seen in children.

- 5% metastasize, usually to regional nodes.

- Rarely, distant osteoblastic metastasis to bone.

- 10-year survival → 70%.

- Cytology often negative, as tumor is covered by mucosa.

- Treatment: surgical resection.

- Gross:
  - Solitary, intrabronchial polypoid mass that may infiltrate bronchial wall.
  - Covered by intact mucosa.
  - Gray-yellow cut surface.
  - Cartilage may be present.

- Microscopy:
  - Nests/cords of uniform, bland cells.

- With central nuclei and moderate granular cytoplasm.
- Prominent vasculature.
- Stroma may be delicate fibrovascular, hyalinized, or exhibit calcification.
- Lymphovascular invasion common.
- Rarely, mitotic figures, rosettes, papillae, endocrine atypia, or melanin.
- Possible paraganglioma look with S100 (+) sustentacular cells.
- May have oncocytic features.

- Positive stains:
  - Keratin, serotonin, chromogranin A and B, synaptophysin, CD56/Leu7, pancreatic polypeptide.

- Negative stains:
  - Mucin, TTF-1.

- Differential diagnosis:
  - Small-cell carcinoma.

Peripheral carcinoid tumor

- Arise in peripheral lung, often beneath the pleura.

- Usually asymptomatic and incidental.

- Excellent prognosis.

- Rare nodal metastasis.

- Usually cured by excision.

- Treatment: lobectomy (as multiple tumors are common).

- Gross:
  - Multiple gray-tan nodules.
  - Non-encapsulated
  - Brown-tan, cut surface.
  - Not associated with a bronchus.

- Microscopy:
  - Disorderly spindle cells resembling smooth muscle.
  - Moderate pleomorphism and mitotic activity.
  - Prominent stroma.
  - Amyloid and melanin often present.

- Positive stains:
  - Congo Red (amyloid), calcitonin.

Atypical carcinoid tumor

- Also called moderately differentiated neuroendocrine carcinoma.
- Resembles a carcinoid but with atypical features.
- More aggressive than typical carcinoid tumors.
- Common nodal metastases.
- 5-year survival → 50–70%.
- Microscopy:
  - Carcinoid tumors with ↑ mitotic activity (2–10 per 10 high-power fields (HPF)).
  - ↑ nuclear pleomorphism.
  - Foci of necrosis.
- Positive stains:
  - More intense neuroendocrine staining than small-cell carcinoma; also (+) for pancreatic polypeptide.
- Negative stains:
  - TTF.

Adenoid cystic carcinoma

- May arise from submucus bronchial glands.
- Usually in large bronchi; may involve the trachea.
- Frequent metastases to regional lymph nodes and lung parenchyma.
- Prolonged course, but overall prognosis is poor.
- Treatment: radiation therapy (palliative).
- Gross:
  - Large, polypoid, intrabronchial mass.
  - May grow subepithelially along the bronchi.
- Positive stains:
  - Variable ductal and myoepithelial phenotype.
  - Cytokeratin, vimentin, C-kit, smooth-muscle actin, calponin, S-100, P63, GFAP.
- Differential diagnosis:
  - Basaloid carcinoma with adenoid cystic carcinoma-like pattern.

Epithelial–myoepithelial carcinoma

[Doganay L, *Arch Pathol Lab Med* **127**: e177–e180, 2003]

- Arises from submucosal bronchial glands.
- Mimics the similar salivary gland tumor.
- Very rare.
- Ages 40–69 years.
- Low-grade malignancy.
- Long interval to recurrence or metastasis.
- Gross:
  - Intraluminal bronchial polypoid mass.
  - May invade pulmonary parenchyma.
- Microscopy:
  - Well-circumscribed mass.
  - Pushing margin.
  - Duct-like structures: inner epithelial cells/outer clear myoepithelial cells.
  - No myxoid/chondroid stroma.
  - No perineural invasion.
- Positive stains:
  - Epithelial cells (keratin, EMA, myoepithelial cells), S100, smooth muscle actin (SMA).
- Negative stains:
  - HMB45.
- Differential diagnosis:
  - Mucoepidermoid carcinoma.
  - Pleomorphic adenoma.
  - Adenoid cystic carcinoma with a tubular pattern.
  - Myoepithelioma.
  - Metastatic epithelial–myoepithelial carcinoma.
  - Myoepithelial carcinoma.
  - Metastatic clear cell carcinoma.
  - Clear cell tumor.
  - Acinic cell carcinoma.

Mucoepidermoid carcinoma

- May arise from submucus bronchial glands.

- Usually in large bronchi.
- May occur in children.
- Low malignant potential with recurrence.
- Rarely aggressive.
- Excellent prognosis after surgical removal.
- Gross:
  - Polypoid growth in major bronchi.
- Microscopy:
  - Low grade or high grade.
  - Mucus secreting, squamous, or intermediate-type cells.
- Differential diagnosis:
  - Adenosquamous carcinoma arising from bronchial epithelium.

Sebaceous carcinoma

- Microscopy:
  - Sebaceous differentiation.
  - Lobulated and infolded architecture.
  - Basaloid cells with sharp cytoplasmic borders.
- Positive stains:
  - Oil red O.
- Negative stains:
  - PAS-diastase, mucicarmine.
- Differential diagnosis:
  - Metastatic tumor.
  - Mucoepidermoid carcinoma.
  - SCC with sebaceous differentiation.

Other tumors

Pleuropulmonary blastoma

- Children < 10 years old.
- Microscopy:
  - Cystic or solid sarcoma.
  - Cysts lined with metaplastic epithelium.

   – Features of chondrosarcoma, leiomyosarcoma, rhabdomyosarcoma, liposarcoma, undifferentiated sarcoma.

Hamartoma

- Also called pulmonary chondroma.
- Benign, predominantly ♂ adults.
- Usually solitary, subpleural.
- Presents as incidental coin lesion, with popcorn pattern of calcification on chest radiograph.
- May present as intrabronchial polypoid mass causing obstruction.
- Gross:
    - ≤ 4 cm.
    - Sharply delineated and lobulated.
    - Glistening cut surface with ill-defined clefts.
- Microscopy:
    - Islands of mature hyaline cartilage, fat, smooth muscle, and clefts lined by respiratory epithelium.
    - Cartilage may be calcified or ossified.
    - Periphery of cartilage may contain immature myxomatous tissue.

Inflammatory myofibroblastic tumor

- Equal sex distribution and all ages.
- Most < 40 years old.
- Most common mesenchymal tumor of childhood.
- Poor prognostic factors:
    - Metastasis.
    - Necrosis > 15% of surface area.
    - Local recurrence.
    - Bizarre giant cells.
    - > 3 mitotic figures/50 HPF.
    - Advanced stage.
    - High cellularity.
    - Poor circumscription.
- Gross:
    - Well circumscribed.

- – Non-encapsulated.
- – Usually solitary, white, firm, parenchymal nodule.
- – 3% bilateral.
- – May have hemorrhage, necrosis, calcification.

- Microscopy:
  - – Plasma cells, lymphocytes, histiocytes, myofibroblasts.
  - – May have vascular proliferation, collagenous or hyalinized stroma, myxoid change, xanthoma cells, hemosiderin.
  - – May resemble nodular fascitis, fibrous histiocytoma, or fibromatosis.

- Positive stains:
  - – Spindle cells: vimentin, smooth-muscle actin, rarely desmin, ALK1.

- Differential diagnosis:
  - – Hemangiopericytoma.
  - – Carcinoid tumor.
  - – Plasmacytoma.
  - – Amyloid tumor.
  - – Metastatic carcinoma.
  - – Tuberculosis.
  - – Organizing pneumonia.
  - – Lipid pneumonia.
  - – Fibrous histiocytoma.
  - – Other spindle cell tumors.
  - – Mycobacterial pseudotumor.

Sclerosing hemangioma

- Predominantly middle age ♀.

- Presents as incidental solitary nodule on chest radiograph.

- Apparently derived from type II pneumocytes.

- Almost always benign.

- 2–4% have nodal metastases that do not appear to affect prognosis.

- Sclerosis and hemorrhage are probably secondary changes.

- Gross:
  - – Well circumscribed and non-encapsulated.
  - – Easily shelled out.
  - – Tan-yellow and may be hemorrhagic.
  - – Usually peripheral lung.

- Microscopy:
  - Two cell type: round stromal cells and surface cells.
  - Round cells:
    - Well-defined border.
    - Central oval bland nuclei.
    - Fine chromatin.
    - No nucleoli.
    - Foamy eosinophilic cytoplasm.
  - Surface cells:
    - Resemble bronchoalveolar epithelium or activated type II penumocytes.
- Focal, mild to marked, atypical in either cell type.
- Frequent hemorrhage and aggregates of histiocytes.
- No/rare granulomatous reaction.
- No/rare mitotic figures.
- No angiolymphatic invasion.
- No necrosis.
- Four patterns:
  - Papillary.
  - Sclerotic.
  - Solid.
  - Hemorrhagic.
- Immunohistochemistry:
  - Round cells:
    - TTF-1, EMA, keratin (–).
  - Surface cells:
    - TTF-1, EMA, keratin, surfactant proteins
- Negative stains (round and surface cells):
  - CEA, S100, smooth-muscle actin, chromogranin, CD34.
- Differential diagnosis:
  - Primary and metastatic carcinoma.
  - Clear cell.
  - Carcinoid tumor.
  - Papillary adenoma.
  - Alveolar adenoma.
  - Epithelioid hemangioendothelioma.
  - Langerhans cell histiocytosis.

Solitary fibrous tumor

- May be intrapulmonary and not pleural.
- Peaks at ages 50–69 years.
- Larger tumors associated with:
  - Hypoglycemia.
  - Pleural effusion.
  - Pulmonary osteoarthropathy.
- Gross:
  - Firm.
  - Rounded and lobulated.
  - Variable cysts, hemorrhage, necrosis.
- Microscopy:
  - Highly variable cellularity.
  - Markedly collagenous stroma.
  - Irregularly distributed, thick-walled vessels.
  - May have myxoid stroma.
  - Often has malignant features.
  - May have malignant fibrous histiocytoma, hemangiopericytoma, fibrosarcoma, or neural patterns.
- Positive stains:
  - CD34, bcl-2, vimentin; variable smooth-muscle actin.
- Differential diagnosis:
  - Sarcomatoid carcinoma.
  - Hemangiopericytoma.
  - Sarcomatoid mesothelioma.
  - Malignant fibrous histiocytoma.
  - Thymoma.
  - Peripheral nerve sheath tumors.

Epitheliod hemangioendothelioma

- 80% ♀, usually young adults and Caucasian.
- Neoplastic, but usually not metastatic.
- Progressive growth, usually remains within thoracic cavity.
- May cause death from respiratory insufficiency.
- Other sites: liver, bone.

- 10% have peripheral eosinophilia.
- Poor prognosis if vascular spread, pleural involvement, severe symptoms.
- Gross:
  - Multiple, round, well-demarcated nodules < 2 cm.
  - Often in lower lung.
  - May spread along pleura or pericardium and resemble mesothelioma.
- Microscopy:
  - Central hyalinized stroma.
  - Eosinophilic amorphous material.
  - May see coagulative necrosis with variable calcification surrounded by thin rim of plump eosinophilic endothelial cells.
  - Clusters fill alveoli, and occasionally bronchioles, arteries, and veins.
  - Nuclei are bland, round/oval, and may have cytoplasmic vacuoles.
  - No/minimal mitoses.
  - Lung architecture preserved.
- Positive stains:
  - Factor VIII, CD31, CD34, Fli variable estrogen receptor (ER) and progesterone receptor (PR).
- Differential diagnosis:
  - Metastatic tumor from liver or other sites.
  - Sclerosing hemangioma.
  - Old granuloma.
  - Organizing infarct.
  - Amyloid nodule.
  - Hamartoma.
  - Hemangioma.
  - Chemodectoma.
  - Mesothelioma.
  - Adenocarcinoma.
  - Angiosarcoma.

Langerhans cell histiocytosis

- Broad age range; usually aged 40 years.
- Strongly associated with smoking.
- 20% with multicentric disease (bone, skin, lymph nodes, spleen, pituitary) have lung involvement.
- 50% of cases involve only lung.

- Associated with pneumothorax, *Pneumocystis carinii* pneumonia.

- Usually lung disease resolves or stabilizes, but 10–20% may progress to respiratory failure.

- Gross:
  - Involves upper lobes.
  - Nodules and cavitary lesions and late honeycombing.
  - Local or diffuse process.

- Microscopy:
  - Interstitial scarring with nodular aggregates of Langerhans cells.
  - Bronchiolocentric distribution.
  - Prominent eosinophils and mesothelial cells.
  - Langerhans cells:
    - Abundant eosinophilic cytoplasm.
    - Grooved nuclei.
    - Indented nuclear membrane.
    - Frequent hemosiderin and necrosis.
    - Alveolar lining cell hyperplasia present.
    - Pigmented alveolar macrophages.
    - Variable vasculitis.
    - Older lesions have fewer eosinophils and more interstitial fibrosis.
    - Sarcomatous variant has significant atypia and mitotic figures.

- Positive stains:
  - CD1a, S100, HLA-DR.

- Differential diagnosis:
  - Eosinophilic pleuritis.
  - Reactive Langerhans cells in inflammatory conditions.
  - Desquamative interstitial pneumonitis.

Benign metastasizing leiomyoma

- Rare.

- Usually ♀ aged 36–64 years.

- Often history of uterine leiomyomas.

- May regress during pregnancy or after oophorectomy.

- May represent a well-differentiated leiomyosarcoma of low malignant potential, metastatic to lung.

- Usually no symptoms, or mild cough and shortness of breath.

- Good prognosis

- Microscopy:
    - Well circumscribed.
    - Single or multiple nodules of smooth muscle.
    - Eosinophilic cytoplasm, oval nuclei, inconspicuous nucleoli.
    - Large, thick-walled vessels.
    - No atypia, no vascular invasion, no mitotic figures.

- Differential diagnosis:
    - Hamartoma.
    - Low-grade leiomyosarcoma.

Clear cell (sugar) tumor

- Rare.

- Wide age range.

- Associated with tuberous sclerosis.

- Occurs in periphery.

- Derived from perivascular epithelioid cells.

- Gross:
    - Small, sharply outlined, red-tan mass.

- Microscopy:
    - Large cells with clear to eosinophilic granular cytoplasm and numerous PAS (+) glycogen granules.
    - Small uniform nuclei.
    - Prominent vasculature.
    - No mitotic figures.

- Positive stains:
    - HMB45, S100 (focal).

- Negative stain:
    - Keratin.

- Differential diagnosis:
    - Carcinoma with clear cell pattern.
    - Metastatic renal cell carcinoma.
    - Metastatic melanoma.
    - Metastatic clear cell sarcoma.

Lymphangioleiomyomatosis

- Rare, unknown etiology, may diffusely involve both lungs.
- Almost always in ♀, usually white and of reproductive age.
- Rare cases in ♂ or postmenopausal ♀ on hormone replacement therapy.
- Associated with tuberous sclerosis.
- May involve mediastinal or periaortic lymph nodes.
- Derived from perivascular epithelioid cells.
- Associated with germline mutation of TSC1 and TSC2.
- Poor prognosis – death due to respiratory failure or cor pulmonale.
- Disease worsened by pregnancy or menstruation, improved post-menopause.
- Gross:
  - Emphysematous-like changes to widespread cystic spaces separated by thick, gray-white septa.
- Microscopy:
  - Cystic air spaces and patchy disordered nodular proliferation of bland smooth muscle around airways, lymphatic system, blood vessels.
  - Proliferating, smooth-muscle cells expand lung parenchyma.
  - Hemosiderin pigment is common.
- Positive stains:
  - HMB45, ER, PR.
- Differential diagnosis:
  - Metastatic endometrial sarcoma.
  - Benign metastasizing leiomyoma.
  - Idiopathic pulmonary hemosiderosis.
  - Micronodular pneumocyte hyperplasia.

Micronodular pneumocyte hyperplasia

- Associated with tubular sclerosis.
- May coexist with lymphangioleiomyomatosis.
- Usually ♀ with shortness of breath.
- Considered a hamartoma.

- 5-year survival is 50%.
- Microscopy:
  - Pleomorphic, large lymphoid cells, usually non-cleaved.
  - Necrosis, and pleural and vascular involvement are common.
- Positive stains:
  - CD20, CD79a.
- Negative stains:
  - CD3, CD5.
- Differential diagnosis:
  - Undifferentiated carcinoma.
  - Variants of Hodgkin's lymphoma.
  - Anaplastic, large-cell lymphoma.
  - Rarely, germ cell tumor.

Metastatic tumors to lung

- Lung is a common site of metastases.
- Usually multiple, bilateral, sharply outlined, rapidly growing.
- More pleomorphic and necrotic than lung primaries.
- TTF-1 (–).
- Often multiple, discrete nodules in periphery of lung.
- Lymphangitis carcinomatosa.
- Nodular metastases:
  - Breast.
  - Gastrointestinal tract.
  - Kidney.
  - Sarcoma.
  - Melanoma.
- Lymphangitis carcinomatosis:
  - Stomach.
  - Breast.
  - Choriocarcinoma.
  - Pancreas.
  - Prostate.
- Central cavitation:
  - SCC of upper aerodigestive tract.

- Colonic adenocarcinoma.
- Leiomyosarcoma.

- Intrabronchial masses:
  - Breast.
  - Kidney, colon.

- Tumor emboli:
  - Breast.
  - Stomach.
  - Liver.
  - Choriocarcinoma.

- Lepidic pattern:
  - Colon.
  - Pancreas.

Adenocarcinoma vs mesothelioma

[Ordonez NG, *Am J Surg Pathol* **27**: 1031–1051, 2003]

- Difficult to distinguish if adenocarcinoma does not produce mucin.

- Stains recommended to differentiate between these two tumors:
  - Calretinin.
  - Cytokeratin 5/6.
  - WT1.
  - CEA.
  - MOC31.
  - B72.3.
  - Ber-EP4.
  - BG8.

- Stains specific for <u>adenocarcinoma</u> vs mesothelioma:
  - Ber-EP4 (100% vs 18%).
  - MOC31 (100% vs 8%).
  - BG8 (96% vs 7%).
  - CEA (88% vs 0%).
  - B72.3 (84% vs 0%).
  - TTF-1 (74% vs 0%).
  - CD15/LeuM1 (72% vs 0%).

- Stains specific for <u>mesothelioma</u> vs adenocarcinoma:
  - Calretinin (100% vs 8%).
  - Cytokeratin 5/6 (100% vs 2%).

- WT1 (93% vs 0%).
- Thrombomodulin (77% vs 14%).

- Stains frequently positive in both tumors:
  - EMA.
  - E-cadherin.
  - HBME.
  - CD44S mesothelin.
  - Vimentin.

CHAPTER 7

Surgery in non-small-cell lung cancer

Types of surgical procedure

[Van Schil PE. *Lung Cancer* **34**: S127–S132, 2001]

Standard procedures

- Pneumonectomy.
- Lobectomy.
- Bilobectomy.

Atypical, conservative, or parenchyma-sparing operations

- Proximal.
  - Bronchotomy.
  - Rotating bronchoplasty.
  - Bronchial or tracheal wedge excision.
  - Bronchial or tracheal sleeve resection.
- Distal.
  - Segmentectomy.
  - Wedge excision.

Extended procedures (lung + other structure)

- Pericardium (intrapericardial pneumonectomy).
- Diaphragm.

- Chest wall (ribs, vertebrae).
- Superior sulcus (Pancoast tumor).

Pneumonectomy

- Removal of an entire lung.
- There have been no randomized trials comparing pneumonectomy vs lobectomy.
- Recommended when the primary tumor or lymph node (LN) involvement extends to the proximal bronchus or proximal pulmonary artery, or crosses the major fissure such that a complete resection is possible only by pneumonectomy.

Lobectomy via thoracotomy or video-assisted thoracocoscopy

[Churchill ED, *J Thorac Cardiovasc Surg* **20**: 349–365, 1950]

- Removal of a lung lobe.
- Procedure of choice in early-stage disease, when a complete resection can be accomplished and complete excision can be achieved by lobectomy, thus:
  - Sparing functioning lung.
  - Locoregional recurrence is ↑ and survival is ↓ if < lobectomy is performed.
- [Endo C, *Ann Thorac Cardiovasc Surg* **9**: 283–289, 2003]
  - Vast majority performed via thoracotomy.
  - Typically, cancers <u>not</u> amenable to VATS resection include:
    - Tumors > 5 cm in diameter, T_3 lesions, and those with extensive LN involvement.
  - Several investigators no longer exclude patients with LN metastases or individuals who have received induction therapy.
  - Video-assisted thoracocoscopy (VATS), whenever feasible, can be done with results comparable to those obtained by thoracotomy, according to some authors.

Video-assisted thoracocoscopy and early-stage non-small-cell lung cancer

[Chang MY, *Semin Surg Oncol* **21**: 74–84, 2003]
[Gajra A, *Lung Cancer* **42**: 51–57, 2003]

[Nonaka M, *Am J Clin Oncol* **26**: 499–503, 2003]

- VATS lobectomy is performed with lung isolation and the placement of several 2 cm port sites as well as a 5–8 cm 'utility' incision, through which instruments are placed for hilar dissection

- VATS lung resections are less invasive than those performed by thoracotomy and typically enable patients to return to normal activity sooner than patients undergoing comparable lung resection by thoracotomy.
  - Hospital stay is ↓, postoperative pain is diminished, and chest tubes are removed sooner in patients undergoing VATS procedures than in those undergoing thoracotomy.
  - No apparent late differences in pain or morbidity have been noted in patients undergoing VATS.
  - The adequacy of VATS resection for lung cancer has not been clearly established.

- Reported 4-year survival rate of 70% for patients with stage I lung cancer undergoing VATS resection.
  [McKenna RJ Jr, *Ann Thorac Surg* **66**: 1903–1908, 1998]

- Reported 5-year survival rates of 78% for stage I, 51% for stage II, and 29% for stage III carcinomas; these results are comparable with those for open procedures.
  [Walker WS, *Eur J Cardiothorac Surg* **23**: 397–402, 2003]

- 100 patients with stage IA lung cancer were prospectively randomly assigned to undergo VATS lobectomy or conventional resection.
  [Sugi K, *World J Surg* **24**: 27–31, 2000]
  - Mediastinal lymph node dissections (MLNDs) were performed in all patients.
  - The average size of the tumors in both groups was 2 cm.
  - The 5-year overall survival in the VATS and open lobectomy groups was 90% and 85%, respectively.

- CONCLUSION:
  - Although, in experienced hands, VATS lobectomy appears comparable to conventional lobectomy for the treatment of early-stage disease, the role of VATS in more advanced lung cancer has yet to be determined.
    - Overall, the prognosis of the patient depends on the extent of the pulmonary resection and MLND, and the surgical technique should be that which the surgeon is most competent to perform.

- After resection for stage I and II lung cancer, the 5-year survival rate without recurrence exceeds 50% in stage I disease and 35% in stage II disease.
- In completely resected T_1N_0 tumors, 5-year survival rates exceed 70%, and in some series surpass 80%.

Bilobectomy

- Removal of two lobes on the right side.

- Indicated when a tumor involves the bronchus intermedius.

Laser resection (segmentectomy, wedge resection, precision cautery dissection) vs lobectomy

- The role of these procedures in peripheral T_1N_0 tumors has yet to be fully defined.

- Patients selected for segmentectomy or wedge resections tend to have more impaired pulmonary reserve and to exhibit other significant comorbidities.

- Lung Cancer Study Group.
  [Ginsberg RJ, *Ann Thorac Surg* **60**: 615–623, 1995]
  – In a randomized trial in patients with T_1N_0 NSCLC, on long-term follow-up the locoregional recurrence rate was $3\times \uparrow$ with limited resection vs lobectomy (15% vs 5%).
  – Morbidity, mortality, and pulmonary function were equal in both groups.
  – A marginally significant long-term survival benefit was noted for lobectomy.

- Retrospective review.
  [Warren WH, *J Thorac Cardiovasc Surg* **107**: 1087–1094, 1994]
  – Locoregional recurrence was $\uparrow$ after segmentectomy vs after lobectomy.
  – Difference was primarily seen in stage II carcinomas.
  – No survival difference was observed for T_1N_0 carcinomas resected by lobectomy or segmentectomy.

- Single institution study comparing segmentectomy vs lobectomy for the treatment of T_1N_0 carcinoma in patients with adequate pulmonary reserve for lobectomy.
  [Kodama K, *J Thorac Cardiovasc Surg* **114**: 347–353, 1997]

- – 5-year overall survival, recurrence rates, and lung-cancer-related deaths were comparable in the two treatment groups.
- – Of note, the average tumor diameter was significantly larger in the lobectomy group than in the segmentectomy group (2.29 vs 1.67 cm).

- Comparison of limited resection in 74 patients vs lobectomy in 159 patients for treatment of T_1 (< 2 cm) peripheral lung cancer. [Koike T, *J Thorac Cardiovasc Surg* **125**: 924–928, 2003]
  - – All patients had adequate pulmonary reserve for lobectomy.
  - – No significant differences were noted in 3-year or 5-year survival rates for these individuals.

- Retrospective series reviewed the Mayo Clinic experience pertaining to surgical treatment of 100 patients with lung carcinomas ≤ 1 cm in diameter. [Miller DL, *Ann Thorac Surg* **73**: 1545–1551, 2002]
  - – 75 patients underwent lobectomy or bilobectomy, and 25 underwent segmentectomy or a wedge resection.
  - – Tumor diameters ranged from 3 to 10 mm. Seven patients had LN metastases. Lung-cancer-specific 5-year survival was 85.4%.
  - – Patients undergoing lobectomy had improved survival and fewer recurrences than those undergoing limited resection.

- Although the role of segmentectomy is being reconsidered for NSCLC of ≤ 2 cm, segmentectomies are seldom performed for lung cancer except in patients with compromised lung function

- Lung Cancer Study Group. [Ginsberg RJ, *Ann Thorac Surg* **60**: 615–623, 1995]
  - Prospective multi-institutional randomized trial, 1982–1988.
  - 276 patients with T_1N_0 NSCLC were randomized to lobectomy vs limited resection.
  - Analysis included locoregional and distant recurrence rates, 5-year survival rates, perioperative morbidity and mortality, and late pulmonary function assessment.
  - CONCLUSIONS:
    - – Compared with lobectomy, limited pulmonary resection does not confer improved perioperative morbidity, mortality, or late postoperative pulmonary function.
    - – Because of the higher death rate and locoregional recurrence rate associated with limited resection, lobectomy still must be considered the surgical procedure of choice for patients with peripheral T_1N_0 NSCLC.

- 173 patients with stage I NSCLC underwent either standard lobectomy or a segmental resection; survival and the prevalence of local/regional recurrence were assessed.
  [Warren WH, *J Thorac Cardiovasc Surg* **107**: 1087–1094, 1994]
  - Retrospective non-randomized study, 1980–1988.
  - RESULTS:
    - Although no survival advantage of lobectomy over segmental resection was noted for patients with tumors ≤ 3.0 cm in diameter, a survival advantage was apparent for patients undergoing lobectomy for tumors > 3.0 cm.
    - The rate of local/regional recurrence was 22.7% after segmental resection vs 4.9% after lobectomy.
    - A review of histologic type, original tumor diameter, and segment resected revealed no risk factors that were predictive of recurrence.
  - CONCLUSIONS:
    - Lobectomy is the preferred surgical procedure for patients with stage I tumors > 3.0 cm in diameter.
    - Because the rate of local/regional recurrence was high after segmental resection, diligent follow-up of these patients is mandatory.

- 184 patients with small peripheral NSCLC were operated on during the period 1993–1996.
  [Takizawa T, *J Thorac Cardiovasc Surg* **118**: 536–541, 1999]
  - Segmentectomy and lobectomy were performed on 48 and 133 good-risk patients, respectively.
  - The aim of this study was to compare the pulmonary function after a segmentectomy with that after a lobectomy for small peripheral carcinoma of the lung.
  - RESULTS:
    - 12 months after surgery, the segmentectomy and lobectomy groups had forced vital capacities of 2.67 ± 0.73 and 2.57 ± 0.59 l, which were calculated to be 94.9 ± 10.6% and 91.0 ± 13.2%, respectively, of the preoperative values.
    - The segmentectomy and lobectomy groups had postoperative 1-second forced expiratory volumes of 1.99 ± 0.63 l and 1.95 ± 0.49 l, which were calculated to be 93.3 ± 10.3% and 87.3 ± 14.0% of the preoperative values, respectively.
  - CONCLUSIONS:
    - Pulmonary function after a segmentectomy for a good-risk patient is slightly better than that after a lobectomy.

- However, segmentectomy should still be the surgical procedure of choice for poor-risk patients because of the difficulty of excluding patients with metastatic LNs from the candidates for the procedure.

In summary

- Current data do not clearly support the routine use of limited resection for peripheral stage I lung cancer in patients who are candidates for lobectomy.

- Nevertheless, anatomic segmentectomy may be reasonable for individuals with peripheral tumors < 3 cm in diameter that exhibit no endobronchial extension or intrapulmonary metastases and do not involve N_1 or N_2 LN stations on the basis of intraoperative staging.

- The role of limited resection for very small (< 1 cm) tumors, such as those detected by computerized tomography (CT) screening methods, needs to be evaluated in well-designed, prospective studies.

Sublobar resection with adjuvant intraoperative brachytherapy

- [El-Sherif A, *Surg Oncol* **14**(1): 27–32 (review), 2005].
  Adjuvant intraoperative brachytherapy as an alternative to external beam radiation following sublobar resection.

- [R. Santos, *Surgery* **134**: 691–697, 2003]
  - Iodine-125 (^{125}I) implants are used, fashioned, and placed on the staple line. The ^{125}I seeds are embedded in vicryl sutures.
  - ^{125}I sutures are sewn onto a piece of polyglyconate mesh (Ethicon Inc, Somerville, NJ) at an appropriate spacing to achieve a prescribed dose of 10,000–12,000 cGy to a depth of 0.5 cm.
  - The ^{125}I implant is then secured by the thoracic surgeon over the staple line with an approximate 2 cm margin.
  - The mesh is secured to the lung using interrupted 3.0 silk sutures.

- The advantage of brachytherapy is that it provides a means of delivering radiation in a more uniform manner, with 100% patient compliance and in the same setting as the lung resection.

- A study from Pittsburgh compared local recurrence rates in 98 patients undergoing sublobar resection with brachytherapy to 102 patients undergoing sublobar resection alone.

- RESULTS:
  - No differences in surgical mortality, distal recurrence, or survival.
  - Local recurrence was significantly ↓ from 18.6% to 2% in patients who had adjuvant brachytherapy.

- Brachytherapy in 33 high-risk patients, primarily after wedge resection. [Lee W, *Ann Thorac Surg* **75**(1): 237–242, 242–243 (discussion), 2003]
  - RESULTS:
    - The local recurrence rate → 6.1%.
    - Similar to the 6.4% reported after lobectomy in the Lung Cancer Study Group study.

- Z4032.
  - As a result of these pilot studies, the American College of Surgeons Oncology Group will soon open a study (Z4032) using adjuvant brachytherapy for high-risk patients with T_1N_0 NSCLC to confirm these findings in a multicenter setting.

Bronchoplastic procedures

- [Jensik RJ, The extent of resection for localized lung cancer: segmental resection. In: Kittle CF (ed.), *Current Controversies in Thoracic Surgery*. Philadelphia, PA, WB Saunders, p. 175, 1986]
  - 296 patients.
  - Estimated 5-year survival rate 52%.
  - Operative mortality rate 1%.
  - Local recurrence rate 12%.
  - In proximally situated tumors (T_3) for which a pneumonectomy may be required for a total excision, lung-conserving operations using bronchoplastic procedures (to preserve uninvolved lobes, e.g. sleeve lobectomy) have equivalent results to the more extensive pneumonectomy and should be employed when possible, even when the proximal pulmonary artery is involved.

Mediastinal lymphadenectomy

[Gajra A, *J Clin Oncol* **21**: 1029–1034, 2003]
[Izbicki JR, *Br J Surg* **81**: 229–235, 1994]

- The role of mediastinal lymphadenectomy as part of the surgical procedure remains controversial.

- Some investigators feel that aggressive LN dissections improve the accuracy of the staging and survival.

- ECOG 3590.
  [Keller SM, *Ann Thorac Surg* **70**: 358–366, 2000]
  - 373 patients with stage II and stage IIIA NSCLC were randomly assigned to undergo pulmonary resection with either systematic sampling or complete ipsilateral MLND.
  - Although the percentages of patients with N_1 and N_2 disease were comparable in the two groups, more patients were found to have multilevel N_2 disease in the MLND group.
  - Patients who underwent MLND had statistically longer survival compared with those evaluated by systematic sampling (64 vs 25 months, respectively);
  - The survival advantage in the MLND group was restricted to individuals with right-sided cancer (possibly due to the lack of complete resection of L_2 and L_4 LN stations in the MLND group).
- A randomized trial involving 471 evaluable patients.
  [Wu Y, *Lung Cancer* **36**: 1–6, 2002]
  - There was a statistically significant improvement in survival of patients with stage I, II, and IIIA NSCLC after pulmonary resection with MLND compared to those undergoing lung resection with mediastinal LN sampling.
- In light of the fact that, in experienced hands, MLND does not significantly ↑ the time for surgery or morbidity, it is reasonable to consider complete ipsilateral MLND dissection as the standard of care in all lung cancer resections until unequivocal data indicate appropriate alternatives.
- A small randomized trial comparing mediastinal lymphadenectomy to mediastinoscopy plus intraoperative LN sampling showed no difference in survival, locoregional recurrence, or accuracy of the two staging procedures as applied to stage I or II lung cancer.
- A large phase III trial is underway in North America to address this issue.

Radiofrequency ablation

- Only 15% of lung cancer patients are candidates for surgery because most of them present with already advanced disease or have too many comorbidities.
- Minimally invasive therapies using thermal energy sources (radiofrequency, cryoablation, focused ultrasound, laser, and microwave) have emerged in the last decade.

- Radiofrequency ablation (RFA) is the best developed of these therapies.

- RFA is safe and technically highly successful in terms of initial ablation.

- RFA uses needle electrodes to deliver an alternating current that generates ionic agitation, localized frictional tissue heating, and cell death.

- Ultrasound is the preferred technique for electrode placement, but where ultrasound is not possible (e.g. in lung ablation or in ultrasound occult liver tumors) then CT or magnetic resonance imaging (MRI) are used.

- The efficacy of ablation is assessed using contrast-enhanced CT or MRI.
  - Absence of enhancement denotes the area of necrosis.
  - Thermal techniques result in coagulation necrosis and an 'instantaneous thermal fixation' effect.
  - Tissue architecture is preserved, routine histologic stains are misleading, and enzymatic assays are required to establish tissue non-viability.

- RFA can be equally well applied to small lung tumors, either primary or secondary.

- The ideal RFA candidate is a small, peripherally located tumor in a patient who is not suitable for conventional treatment.

- Long-term local control or complete necrosis rates drop considerably when tumors are > 3 cm in size, although repeat ablations can be performed.

- Patients with lung metastases tend to fare better, in terms of local control, with RFA than do those with primary lung carcinoma, but it is unclear if this is related to smaller tumor size at time of treatment, lesion size uniformity, and sphericity with lung metastases, or to differences in the patterns of the pathologic spread of disease.

- Centrally placed tumors carry the additional risk of collateral damage and the ↑ likelihood that adjacent cooling blood vessels may protect tumor cells and result in an ↑ recurrence rate.
  [Suh R, *Oncology (Williston Park)* **19**(11 Suppl 4): 12–21, 2005]

- Several hundred treatments have been performed worldwide, a sufficient number to develop a reasonable safety profile.

- The complication rate is very similar to that seen following percutaneous lung biopsy.
  [Steinke K, *Ann Surg Oncol* **11**: 207–212, 2004]

- Pneumothorax rates are ~ 40%, with only 10–15% requiring drainage or tube insertion.
- The pleural effusion rate is similar at 10%.

- Treatments can be performed under conscious sedation as an overnight or day-case procedure.

- CT guidance is required and CT fluoroscopy is useful.

- Successful ablation is denoted by the development of a ground-glass shadowing that completely encompasses the tumor.
  - Initial consolidation should be larger than the original tumor and then shrink over time, such that only a linear scar is visible at 12 months in 33% of successfully treated tumors.

- Another useful CT feature, which denotes successful ablation, is the absence of enhancement within the consolidated area.

- Ablation of 32 tumors in 30 patients, 26 of whom had primary bronchogenic carcinoma.
  [Lee JM, *Radiology* **230**: 125–134, 2003]
  - Complete ablation was achieved in all six tumors < 3 cm in diameter, and mean survival for this subgroup was 19.7 months vs 8.7 months for the remainder.

- Although several authors have performed percutaneous biopsies in order to detect persistent or recurrent cancer, there are no guidelines regarding timing of biopsy in the post-RFA setting, and there are no data on its accuracy.
  - Therefore, it is difficult to determine the true clinical efficacy of RFA, especially as reported follow-up tends to be short and some recurrences may go undetected.

- A pilot study represents the largest experience with an ablate and resect model in patients with resectable primary NSCLC.
  [Nguyen CL, *Chest* **128**(5): 3507–3511, 2005]
  - 10 patients with stage I or II NSCLC accrued over 2002–2003.
  - RFA was performed through a standard thoracotomy followed by conventional lobectomy and LN dissection.
  - Gross inspection and routine histologic staining could not reliably identify the 'immediately ablated' tissue.
  - Using the nicotinamide adenine dinucleotide (NADH) supravital staining technique, the treated areas from seven of the eight tumors (87.5%) demonstrated > 80% non-viability (100% non-viability was noted in the treated areas from three of the eight tumors).

- No bleeding or thermal complications were noted at the time of RFA, and none of the patients had skin burns at the electrode dispersive pad sites.
- CONCLUSIONS:
  - RFA of primary NSCLC is feasible and can be performed safely in the setting of an open thoracotomy.
  - Complete tumor cell necrosis, as determined by supravital staining, was noted in the treated areas from three of eight tumors (37.5%). Such complete ablation was observed in the treated areas from smaller tumors (< 2 cm), whereas the treated areas from larger tumors demonstrated incomplete ablation.
  - Additional investigation with histopathologic correlation is needed to assess fully the long-term efficacy of RFA for NSCLC.

- Should future studies consistently confirm complete tumor cell necrosis on histopathologic analysis, RFA may become an alternative treatment for T_1N_0 NSCLC, small pulmonary metastases, and local recurrence in patients who either refuse surgery or who are considered poor surgical candidates.

- Although in the study the success rate of ablating lesions that were < 2 cm was only 50%, results of other studies suggest that RFA is more effective for smaller tumors.
  [Lee JM, *Radiology* **230**: 125–134, 2003]
  [Akeboshi M, *J Vasc Interv Radiol* **15**: 463–470, 2004]
  [Herrera LJ, *J Thorac Cardiovasc Surg* **125**: 929–937, 2003]

- A retrospective report on 493 patients undergoing ablation of pulmonary nodules from seven centers around the world.
  [Steinke K, *Anticancer Res* **24**: 339–343, 2004]
  - The main focus was primarily a discussion of perioperative mortality and morbidity.
  - The authors concluded that RFA was safe, with negligible mortality, little morbidity, short hospital stay, and a gain in quality of life.
  - LIMITATIONS OF THE STUDY:
    - Few follow-up data exist regarding efficacy.
    - Most patients with solitary pulmonary nodules, or oligometastatic disease to the lungs, will be asymptomatic, and as such are unlikely to demonstrate a gain in quality of life after treatment.
    - No data were presented that support the authors' claim that quality of life improves following RFA.

- 33 lung tumors in 18 patients (12 ♂, 6 ♀) were treated with RFA.
  [Herrera LJ, *J Thorac Cardiovasc Surg* **125**: 929–937, 2003]

- Tumors included metastatic carcinoma ($n = 8$), sarcoma ($n = 5$), and lung cancer ($n = 5$).
- Mean age → 60 years (range 27–95 years).
- Thoracic surgeons performed RFA minithoracotomy ($n = 5$) or used CT-guided percutaneous methods ($n = 13$) in patients under general anesthesia in the operating room.
- Mean length of stay → 3 days (range 1–7 days).
- SIDE EFFECTS:
  - Procedure-related pneumothorax in 7/13 (53.8%) percutaneous procedures, delayed pneumothorax (1/18), pneumonitis/pneumonia (4/18), small pleural effusion (9/18), and transient renal failure (1/18). One death occurred as a result of hemoptysis 19 days after RFA of a central nodule. This patient had also received recent brachytherapy.
- RESULTS:
  - Mean follow-up → 6 months (range 1–14 months).
  - RFA achieved a radiographically determined response in 8/12 (66.6%) patients with treated tumors < 5 cm.
  - Death with progressive metastatic disease occurred in 7/18 (38%) patients during follow-up.
- CONCLUSION:
  - This pilot study demonstrates the feasibility of RFA for small peripheral lung tumors.
  - Larger tumors responded poorly.
  - Additional trials are needed to determine the safety and efficacy of RFA.

Notes:
- The treatment response after RFA is difficult to assess.
  [El-Sherif A, *Surg Oncol* **14**(1): 27–32 (review), 2005]

- A residual mass associated with some degree of scarring is usual after RFA.
  - In some cases this scarring may involve a larger area than the original tumor.

- Positron emission tomography (PET) scans may continue to be (+), making it difficult to assess whether viable tumor or scarring is present.

- Different groups have used different criteria to assess tumor progression at follow-up (modified Response Evaluation Criteria in Solid Tumours (RECIST) criteria or CT densitometry protocols).

- Since the inflammatory changes after RFA have often started to subside by 3 months, the 3-month scan is often more useful as the baseline scan against which local progression can be judged.

- The American College of Surgeons Oncology Group will be using this same approach to assess local control after RFA in a study (Z4033) that is currently being developed.
  - A goal of this study is to establish, in a multicenter setting, a common approach to the treatment and follow-up of ablated nodules.

Stereotactic radiosurgery

- Stereotactic radiosurgery is well established for the treatment of intracranial neoplasms, but its use for lung tumors is novel.

- The preliminary report of a phase I trial states that single-fraction stereotactic radiosurgery is safe and feasible for the treatment of selected lung tumors.
  [Whyte RI, *Ann Thorac Surg* **75**(4): 1097–1101, 2003]

- Stereotactic radiosurgery enables the selective delivery of an intense dose of high-energy radiation to destroy a tumor with precision targeting.

- The improved accuracy is achieved by very precise spatial localization of the tumor and the delivery of multiple cross-fired beams of radiation to converge upon the tumor.

- In many centers this has become the standard treatment for intracranial tumors.

- Unlike in the brain, respiratory motion creates difficulties in the delivery of precise radiation to lung tumors.
  - These respiratory displacements are greatest near the diaphragm, and less near the lung apex and adjacent to the carina.
  - One approach to stereotactic radiosurgery is to utilize breath-holding techniques, sometimes in combination with an abdominal compression device to limit the ability of the diaphragm to move caudally.

- A recent study demonstrated a partial response in 87% and a complete response in 27% of 37 high-risk stage I NSCLC patients after stereotactic radiosurgery.
  - At a median follow-up of 15.2 months local recurrence occurred in 6 (16.2%) patients.
    [Timmerman R, *Chest* **124**: 1946–1955, 2003]

The Cyberknife Stereotactic Radiosurgery System (Accuray, Sunnyvale, CA)

- A system that allows better precision for radiation delivery.

- It consists of a linear accelerator radiation source that is mounted on a robotic arm.

- Through the use of image-guided cameras, which image implanted gold fiducial tumor markers placed adjacent to the tumor, the Cyberknife System precisely locates the tumor in space.

- The addition of the Synchrony™ option enables dynamic radiosurgery during respiration.
  - The Synchrony option records the breathing movements of a patient's chest and combines that information with sequential x-ray pictures of the fiducials to facilitate delivery of radiation at any point during the respiratory cycle.
  - This allows further precision with radiation delivery (reducing normal tissue exposure), and is also more comfortable for patients because of the shorter treatment times compared with the breath-holding techniques.

- In a study of 23 patients using the Cyberknife system, 9 cases were performed with breath-holding techniques and 14 with respiratory gating.
  - Treatment responses were complete in 2, partial in 15, stable in 4, and progressive in 2.

In summary

- RFA and stereotactic radiosurgery are promising techniques that appear to be well tolerated, but long-term follow-up is still needed.

- As the use of RFA and stereotactic radiosurgery for NSCLC becomes more prevalent, further studies will be required to compare and determine the appropriate use of each modality, as well as to obtain information regarding the long-term effectiveness, quality of life, and cost-effectiveness of these two techniques.

- RFA and stereotactic radiosurgery are new, minimally invasive, therapies that provide local control of cancers.

- Until further studies are available, these procedures should be offered only to those patients who are at ↑ risk for any form of resection.

Surgical morbidity and mortality in non-small-cell lung cancer

[Delauriers J, *Can J Surg* **32**: 335–339, 1989]

- The most common complications after resectional surgery are cardio-pulmonary problems, especially supraventricular arrhythmias and respiratory failure.

- Lung Cancer Study Group.
  [Ginsberg RJ, *J Thorac Cardiovasc Surg* **86**: 654–658, 1983]
  - ~ 1,200 patients at seven participating centers were evaluated for 30-day surgical mortality over the period 1979–1981.
  - The overall 30-day mortality rate of 3.75 appears to be a reasonable estimate for resectional surgery in lung cancer.

- Pneumonectomies should carry a risk of < 7%, lobectomies < 3%, and lesser resections (segmental or wedge) < 2%.

Surgical treatment of non-small-cell lung cancer based on TNM stage

- In general, surgery is the best treatment modality for patients whose lung cancers are limited to the hemithorax and can be totally encompassed by excision.

- In stage I and stage II disease, when the tumor has not extended beyond the bronchopulmonary LNs, complete (R_0) resections are almost always feasible.

- Currently, there is controversy regarding the management of N_2 disease. Ipsilateral N_2 mediastinal LN involvement, despite being potentially resectable, typically portends limited survival after resection alone.
  - Because of this, pathologic staging of the mediastinum is critical when determining the treatment and prognosis for individuals with locally advanced lung cancer.

- Patients in whom N_2 disease is identified preoperatively have a much poorer prognosis than do individuals with occult N_2 disease discovered only at the time of thoracotomy (5-year survival rates of < 10% vs 30%, respectively).

- By virtue of incontrovertible evidence of contralateral (N_3) LN metastases, or invasion of vital structures such as carina, heart, or great vessels (T_4), or the presence of a malignant pleural effusion (T_4), stage IIIB disease typically is inoperable.

- Similarly, lung cancer that has metastasized to distant organs (stage IV disease) is generally incurable by surgery.

- Occasionally, individuals with solitary brain or adrenal gland metastases may achieve long-term survival after resection of the primary and metastatic lesions.

Surgical treatment of stage I and stage II disease

- Stage I is defined as a T_1 (< 3 cm) or T_2 (> 3 cm) tumor in the parenchyma of the lung, > 2 cm away from the carina, and not invading the chest wall or parietal pleura.
  - Patients who have malignant LNs or distant metastasis are not included. Thus, the TNM classification is either $T_1N_0M_0$ or $T_2N_0M_0$.

- If the patient is a surgical candidate, the current treatment for stage I lung cancer is surgery.

- The surgical procedure of choice, as mentioned above, is a lobectomy, or pneumonectomy with mediastinal LN sampling.

- 5-year survival rate ranges from 71% for stage IA to 57% for stage IB.

- Only 15% of all lung cancers present as stage I disease.

- Stage II is defined as a T_1 tumor with N_1 (hilar LN involvement) and no distant metastasis, or a T_3 tumor with no nodal or distant metastasis ($T_3N_0M_0$).
  - Stage II is further divided into stage IIA (T_1N_1) and IIB (T_2N_1 and T_3N_0), due to differences in survival between the two subgroups.

- Surgical treatment remains the treatment of choice for stage II lung cancer.
  - If the tumor is T_3N_0, the surgery of choice is en bloc resection of the tumor and the chest wall.

- The 5-year survival rate for stage IIA is 52–57%, and that for stage IIB is 24–42%.

- Stage IIA is quite uncommon, representing 1–5% of lung cancer patients treated surgically, while stage IIB represents ~ 15% of surgically treated patients.

T_3N_0 tumors

[Downey RJ, *Ann Thorac Surg* **68**: 188–193, 1999]

- Lung cancers invading the chest wall, diaphragm, or mediastinum are designated T_3 tumors.

- In general, the deeper the invasion, the worse the prognosis.
  - In all instances, it is recommended that these tumors be resected en bloc within all involved structures.

- The prognosis is related to completeness of resection, depth of invasion, and LN status.

- Survival of patients with lung cancer invading the chest wall after resection with curative intent is highly dependent on the extent of nodal involvement and the completeness of resection, and much less so on the depth of chest wall invasion.

- 3,937 patients with NSCLC underwent resection at the National Cancer Center Hospital, Tokyo, from 1962 to 1986.
  [Naruke E, *Ann Thorac Surg* **46**: 603–610, 1988]
  - Outcomes: 5-year survival of patients who had pulmonary resection with and without MLND.
  - 426 patients (25.8%) with N_0M_0 disease.
  - Of these, 345 underwent pulmonary resection with MLND.
  - 5-year survival in this group was 15.9%.
  - In the 81 patients who did not undergo MLND, the 5-year survival was 6.7%.

- The role of MLND as part of the surgical procedure when hilar or mediastinal nodes are uninvolved is under debate.

- The proponents of complete ipsilateral or bilateral MLND argue that complete removal of the mediastinal LNs improves survival.
  - Certainly, this dissection provides the best possible surgical staging by removing all draining LNs, which can then be analyzed pathologically for metastatic involvement.

- Tumors within 2 cm of the carina can be resected by pneumonectomy; however, preservation of distal normal lung, using sleeve resection of main bronchi, is preferred.
  [Martini N. In: Hoogstraten B, Addis BJ, Hansen HH, et al. (eds), *Current Treatment of Cancer, Lung Tumors*. Heidelberg, Springer-Verlag, p. 111, 1988]
  - In the absence of nodal disease, a 5-year survival rate of 35% can be expected.

Stage IIIA disease

[Orlowski TM, *Lung Cancer* **34**: S137–S143, 2001]

- Patients with stage T_3N_1 disease usually undergo surgical resection, but many patients with N_2 disease are disqualified from surgical treatment due to negative prognostic factors.

- Negative prognostic factors compromise:
  - Metastases to upper paratracheal, anterior paratracheal, and subcarinal LNs.
  - Metastases to multiple mediastinal LNs.
  - Occurrence of the so-called 'bulky disease'.
  - Capsular LN invasion.

- The occurrence of one of these negative prognostic factors disqualifies the patient with N_2 disease from radical surgical treatment.

- Patients with unresectable stage IIIA or IIIB NSCLC have traditionally been treated with radiotherapy alone.
  [Arriagada R, *Proc Am Soc Clin Oncol* **16**: 446a (abstract), 1997]
  - Only 5–10% of patients survived beyond 5 years.
  - Distant disease progression (outside the radiation field) occurs in up to 70% of patients, and reflects the presence of systemic micrometastases at the time of initial therapy.

- Stage IIIB disease encompasses patients with a T_4 or an N_3 lesion, both of which are usually considered unresectable.

- A large retrospective study of patients with surgically resected stage IIIB disease.
  [Naruke T, *J Thorac Cardiovasc Surg* **96**: 440–447, 1988]
  - 5-year overall survival rate $\rightarrow$ 6%.
  - 5-year survival $\rightarrow$ 8% in 104 selected patients after resection of a T_4 lesion (the carina and trachea, the heart and great vessels, the esophagus or vertebral body).

- Although primary lung cancer invading the carina is generally considered unresectable, pneumonectomy with tracheal sleeve resection and direct reanastomosis of the trachea to the contralateral main stem bronchus can be accomplished, with reported 5-year survival rates approaching 20%.

[Burt ME, *Surg Clin North Am* **67**: 987–1000, 1987]
[Darteville P, *J Thorac Cardiovasc Surg* **94**: 361, 1987]
- There are case reports of resection of tumors invading the superior vena cava.

- In a retrospective analysis of 18 patients with superior vena cava invasion at Memorial Sloan Kettering Cancer Center (MSKCC), there were no 5-year survivors after resection.

[Choi NC, *Lung Cancer* **18**(Suppl 1): 76 (abstract), 1997]
[Rendina EA, *J Thorac Cardiovasc Surg* **117**: 225–233, 1999]

- The exact role of adjuvant radiotherapy or chemotherapy in T_4 or N_3 tumors is unclear, with very few patients to study.
  - Neoadjuvant and combined modality therapy probably offers the best approach.
  - In one study, 63% of patients underwent a complete resection, and overall survival at 4 years was 19.5%.

- Note: The combined modality role of therapy that includes radiation and chemotherapy is addressed in Chapter 10.

Surgery in stage IV lung cancer

Metastasis (M_1) to lung

- It can be difficult to differentiate between a second primary lung cancer and a metastasis in synchronous lung lesions or among local recurrence, a new primary lung cancer, and a pulmonary metastasis from a previously resected lung cancer.

- A second or recurrent lung lesion is considered a metastasis if the histology is identical to that of the primary tumor and the lesion occurs in the opposite lung or a non-contiguous area of the ipsilateral lung.

- The presence of satellite nodules discovered at surgery, clearly separated from the primary tumor but with identical histologic characteristics, is a poor prognostic factor.
  [Deslauriers J, *J Thorac Cardiovasc Surg* **97**: 504–512, 1989]
  - In patients with satellite nodules from all stages of lung cancer, 5-year survival was 21.6%, compared to 44% if no nodules were present.
  - The mechanism of tumor dissemination in the lung is not well known, but metastases may develop as a result of airborne or hematogenous spread from a primary bronchogenic carcinoma.
  - The present TNM staging system fails to classify these synchronous lung lesions specifically.

- If a solitary synchronous lesion is discovered in a different lobe from the primary tumor, both lesions should be resected whenever possible.

Metastasis (M$_1$) to brain

[Magilligan DJ, *Ann Thorac Surg* **42**: 360–364, 1986]
[Figlin RA, *N Engl J Med* **318**: 1300–1305, 1988]
[Martini N, *Ann Thorac Surg* **42**: 357–358, 1986]
[Patchell RA, *N Engl J Med* **322**: 494–500, 1990]
[Harpole D, *Proc Am Soc Clin Oncol* **15**: 382, 1996]

- Brain metastases constitute more than 25% of all observed recurrences in patients with resected NSCLC, and are seen with greater frequency at autopsy.

- In a review by the Lung Cancer Study Group, the brain was the sole site of first recurrence in only 6.4% of patients with completely resected NSCLC, but accounted for approximately 20% of all recurrences.

- Nearly half of patients with brain metastases have solitary lesions on CT scan.

- Corticosteroids and whole-brain irradiation can offer effective palliation of symptoms, but only modestly ↑ survival up to 6 months.

- A synchronous or metachronous solitary brain metastasis can be treated, whenever possible, by surgical resection, with 5-year survival rates of 10–20%.
  - Surgical excision of a brain metastasis followed by radiation has been shown to be superior to whole-brain radiotherapy alone in prolonging median survival (9.2 vs 3.4 months), in preventing local recurrence, and in providing a better quality of life.
  - Median survival (40 vs 15 weeks) and duration of functional independence (38 vs 8 weeks) were significantly higher in the combined surgery plus radiation arm.

- A resurgence of interest in the use of high-dose three-dimensional conformal radiation therapy (3D CRT) or stereotactic radiosurgery in managing solitary brain metastases has followed early results suggesting equivalence of this approach to surgery.

- MSKCC series.
  [Mandell L, *Cancer* **58**: 641–649, 1986]
  - 104 patients with NSCLC were treated with surgery and radiation ($n = 35$) or radiation alone ($n = 69$).
  - Median survival → 18 months for the combined therapy group vs 4 months for the radiation-alone group.

Metastasis (M$_1$) to the adrenal gland

[Allard P, *Cancer* **66**: 457–462, 1990]
[Twomey P, *JAMA* **248**: 581–583, 1982]
[Raviv G, *J Surg Oncol* **43**: 123–124, 1990]
[Reyes L, *J Surg Oncol* **44**: 32–34, 1990]

- Adrenal metastases from bronchogenic carcinoma are found in ~ 1/3 of patients at autopsy.

- Routine preoperative upper abdominal CT scanning reveals an adrenal mass in ~ 10% of patients.
  - In selected patients, excision of the primary lung tumor and of an isolated adrenal metastasis may improve survival.

- The ultimate role of such an approach in the context of multimodal therapy has yet to be defined.

Neoadjuvant therapy for non-small-cell lung cancer

- Can be chemotherapy, or concurrent chemotherapy and radiation.

Uses of neoadjuvant therapy

- Neo-adjuvant therapy is used to:
  - Stop or eliminate micrometastatic disease.
  - Determine sensitivity to chemotherapy.
  - In down-staging, thereby improving resectability.

Randomized trials

- Controversial due to mixed results.

- Small population size.

- Older chemotherapy agents used in most trials.

Neoadjuvant chemotherapy trials with negative results

- Randomized phase II trial of preoperative chemotherapy vs surgery alone.
  [Dautzenberg B, *Cancer* **65**(11): 2435–2441, 1990]
  - 26 patients with stage I–III non-small-cell lung cancer (NSCLC).
  - Randomized:
    - Group I (PCV group): two preoperative courses of cisplatin 100 mg/m^2, cyclophosphamide 600 mg/m^2 and vindesine

3 mg/m^2 (PCV) chemotherapy, surgery, and two postoperative courses of PCV chemotherapy.
  – Group II (surgery group): immediate surgery.
- RESULTS:
  – A response was observed in 5 patients, and progressive disease was observed in 4 patients with PCV, leading to a cancellation of surgery in two of them.
- CONCLUSION:
  – No difference in median survival (21 vs 23 months).

- Phase III comparison of best local regional therapy with or without chemotherapy for stage IIIA NSCLC.
  [Elias AD, *Proc Am Soc Clin Oncol* **16**: 448a (abstract), 1997]
  - N$_2$ by mediastinoscopy.
  - Trial closed due to poor accrual (57 patients).
  - CONCLUSION:
    – No difference in survival (19 vs 23 months in surgical group).

- Comparative trial on induction chemotherapy followed by surgery or immediate surgery for stage III NSCLC.
  [Yoneda S, *Proc Am Soc Clin Oncol* **14**: 367 (abstract), 1995]
  - Phase III randomized clinical trial.
  - 83 patients stage IIIA and IIIB.
  - ~ 50% were stage IIIB (technically unresectable).
  - Chemotherapy included cisplatin and vindesine.
  - CONCLUSION:
    – No difference. Median survival of 14 months for chemotherapy vs 15 months for surgery.

Neoadjuvant chemotherapy trials with positive results

- Randomized trial of neoadjuvant therapy for NSCLC.
  [Pass HI, *Ann Thorac Surg* **53**(6): 992–998, 1992]
  - 27 patients with stage IIIA (N$_2$) NSCLC.
  - Randomized:
    – Group I (13 patients): preoperative etoposide/cisplatin (EP) chemotherapy, surgery, and postoperative EP.
    – Group II (14 patients): surgery, postoperative mediastinal radiation therapy (XRT) (54–60 Gy).
  - EP therapy: cisplatin 80 mg/m^2 on day 1 and etoposide 120 mg/m^2 on days 1–3.

- Median follow-up → 29.9 months for group I; 34.9 months for group II.
- RESULTS:
  - Median survival time:
    - Group I → 28.7 months.
    - Group II → 15.6 months ($p = 0.095$).

- CONCLUSION:
  - Time to recurrence revealed no significant differences between the two groups, but there was a trend towards increased disease-free interval in the EP group (12.7 vs 5.8 months, EP vs XRT).

- Randomized trial comparing perioperative chemotherapy and surgery with surgery alone in resectable stage IIIA NSCLC.
  [Roth JA, *J Natl Cancer Inst* **86**(9): 673–680, 1994]
  - Prospective, randomized study of 60 patients with stage IIIA NSCLC.
  - Patients with $T_3N_0M_0$ disease were included (now stage IIB).
  - Compare *perioperative* chemotherapy and surgery vs surgery alone.
  - 6 cycles of perioperative chemotherapy (cyclophosphamide, etoposide, and cisplatin) and surgery (28 patients), or surgery alone (32 patients).
  - Patients who had documented tumor regression after preoperative chemotherapy received 3 additional cycles of chemotherapy after surgery.
  - RESULTS:
    - After 3 cycles of preoperative chemotherapy, the rate of clinical major response was 35%.
    - Patients treated with perioperative chemotherapy and surgery had an estimated median survival of 64 vs 11 months for surgery alone ($p < 0.008$)
    - The 2- and 3-year survival rates were 60% and 56% for the perioperative chemotherapy patients and 25% and 15% for surgery alone.
  - CONCLUSION:
    - This trial strengthens the validity of using perioperative chemotherapy in the management of patients with resectable stage IIIA NSCLC.

- Randomized trial comparing preoperative chemotherapy plus surgery with surgery alone in patients with NSCLC.
  [Rosell R, *N Engl J Med* **330**(3):153–158, 1994]
  - Randomized clinical trial of 60 patients with stage IIIA NSCLC.

- Surgery alone or three courses of chemotherapy (mitomycin 6 mg/m^2, ifosfamide 3 g/m^2, and cisplatin 50 mg/m^2 q 3 weeks) followed by surgery.
- All patients received mediastinal XRT (50 Gy) after surgery.
- RESULTS:
  - Median survival → 26 months for chemotherapy plus surgery vs 8 months for surgery alone ($p < 0.001$).
  - Median disease-free survival → 20 vs 5 months ($p < 0.001$).
  - Recurrence rate was 56% in the chemotherapy plus surgery group and 74% with surgery alone.
  - Mutated K-ras oncogenes were present in 15% of patients receiving preoperative chemotherapy and 42% among those receiving surgery alone ($p = 0.05$).
- CONCLUSION:
  - Preoperative chemotherapy ↑ median survival in NSCLC.

- Pre-resectional chemotherapy in randomized controlled stage IIIA NSCLC: 7-year assessment.
  [Rosell R, *Lung Cancer* **26**(1): 7–14, 1999]
  - 60 randomized patients.
  - RESULTS:
    - In 30 patients who received pre-resectional chemotherapy the overall median survival was 22 months (95% CI, 13.4 to 30.6).
    - In 30 patients who received surgery alone the overall median survival was 10 months (95% CI, 7.4 to 12.6; $p = 0.005$).
  - CONCLUSION:
    - Preoperative chemotherapy ↑ median survival in NSCLC.

- Phase III trial of neoadjuvant chemotherapy in resectable stage I, II, and IIIA NSCLC.
  [Depierre A, *Proc Am Soc Clin Oncol* **18**: 465a (abstract), 1999]
  [Depierre A, *J Clin Oncol* **20**(1): 247–255, 2002]
  - 355 patients with stage I (T_2N_0), stage II, or stage IIIA NSCLC.
  - Randomize to chemotherapy plus surgery vs surgery alone.
  - 50% were early stage and 50% stage IIIA (40% with N_2 disease).
  - Two cycles of MIP (mitomycin 6 mg/m^2 day 1, ifosfamide 1.5 g/m^2 days 1–3, and cisplatin 30 mg/m^2 days 1–3) were given. Two more cycles of chemotherapy were given to patients that had objective responses.
  - Postoperative XRT (60 Gy) was given to patients with pT_3 or pN_2 disease in both groups.
  - RESULTS:
    - Overall response rate was 64% (11% complete response).

- 94% of the patients underwent resection.
- Median survival was 37 months for preoperative chemotherapy vs 26 months for primary surgery.
- The 3-year survival was 49% and 41% ($p = 0.02$) for chemotherapy and the control group, respectively.
- Subset analysis showed that the benefit is restricted to stage I and II disease ($p = 0.02$).
- No benefit for N_2 disease.
- CONCLUSION:
  - The impressive differences observed in 3- and 4-year survivals were only statistically significant for stage I and stage II disease.

- Bimodality Lung Oncology Team (BLOT): induction chemotherapy before surgery for early-stage NSCLC
  [Pisters KM, *J Thorac Cardiovasc Surg* **119**(3): 429–439, 2000]
  - Phase II trial of 94 patients with stage IB to IIIA NSCLC (no N_2).
  - All patients required negative mediastinoscopy.
  - Paclitaxel 225 mg/m² over 3 hours and carboplatin (AUC = 6) q 21 days for 2 cycles.
  - Three postoperative cycles of chemotherapy were planned for patients undergoing complete resection.
  - RESULTS:
    - 53 of 94 (56%; 95% CI, 46–67) patients had a major objective response, 88 (94%) underwent surgical exploration, and 81 (86%; 95% CI, 78–92) underwent complete resection.
    - The 1-year survival is estimated → 85%.
  - CONCLUSION:
    - Induction chemotherapy with paclitaxel and carboplatin is feasible and produces a high response rate with acceptable morbidity and mortality in early-stage NSCLC.

- Surgery alone or surgery plus preoperative paclitaxel/carboplatin (PC) chemotherapy in early stage NSCLC (Southwest Oncology Group (SWOG) 9900).
  [Pisters K, ASCO Meeting, abstract 23, 2005]
  - Phase III randomized clinical trial of 354 patients, closed early due to positive adjuvant data.
  - Clinical stage T_2N_0, $T_{1-2}N_1$, and T_3N_{0-1} NSCLCs (excluding superior sulcus tumors) were stratified by clinical stage (IB/IIA vs IIB/IIIA).
  - Median age 64 years, 66% ♂, 36% PS 1, 63% T_2N_0, 5% T_1N_1, 19% T_2N_1, 10% T_3N_0, 4% T_3N_1, 31% adenocarcinoma.

- Group I (180 patients): preoperative paclitaxel/carboplatin (paclitaxel 225 mg/m^2 over 3 hours, carboplatin AUC = 6) on day 1 q 3 weeks ×3.
- Group II (174 patients): surgery alone.
- Median follow-up → 28 months.
- 70% stage IB/IIA, 30% stage IIB/IIIA.
- RESULTS:
  - Major radiographic response to paclitaxel/carboplatin was 40%.
  - Progression-free survival (PFS):
    - Preoperative paclitaxel/carboplatin: median 29 months; 1 year, 68%; 2 years 54%.
    - Surgery alone: 20 months; 1 year, 68%; 2 years, 47%.
    - Hazard rate 0.85 (0.63–1.14), $p = 0.26$.
  - Overall survival (OS):
    - Preoperative paclitaxel/carboplatin group: median, 42 months; 1 year, 82%; 2 years, 68%.
    - Surgery alone: mean, 37 months; 1 year, 79%; 2 years, 64%.
    - Hazard rate 0.88 (0.63–1.23), $p = 0.47$.
- SIDE-EFFECTS:
  - Treatment-related deaths during paclitaxel/carboplatin, 3; deaths within 30 days of surgery, 6 in preoperative paclitaxel/carboplatin group and 4 in surgery alone group.
- CONCLUSION:
  - PFS and OS trends favor preoperative paclitaxel/carboplatin.

Neoadjuvant chemotherapy with concurrent radiation therapy

- Concurrent cisplatin/etoposide plus chest XRT followed by surgery for stages IIIA (N$_2$) and IIIB NSCLC (SWOG 8805 Phase II Study). [Albain K, *J Clin Oncol* **13**(8): 1880–1892, 1995]
  - 126 eligible patients (75 stage IIIA (N$_2$) and 51 stage IIIB).
  - Biopsy proof of either positive N$_2$ nodes (IIIA N$_2$) or of N$_3$ nodes or T$_4$ primary lesions (IIIB) was required.
  - Induction → two cycles of cisplatin and etoposide plus concurrent chest XRT to 45 Gy.
  - Resection was attempted if response or stable disease occurred.
  - Chemotherapy plus XRT boost was given if either unresectable disease or positive margins or nodes were found.
  - Median follow-up time → 2.4 years.

- RESULTS:
  - The objective response rate to induction was 59%, and 29% were stable. Resectability was 85% for the stage IIIA group and 80% for the stage IIIB group.
  - There was no survival difference ($p = 0.81$) between stage IIIA (N_2) vs stage IIIB (median survival 13 and 17 months; 2-year survival 37% and 39%; 3-year survival 27% and 24%).
  - The strongest predictor of long-term survival was absence of tumor in the mediastinal nodes at surgery (median survival 30 vs 10 months; 3-year survival 44% vs 18%; $p = 0.0005$).
- SIDE-EFFECTS:
  - Reversible grade 4 toxicity occurred in 13% of patients.
  - There were 13 treatment-related deaths (10%).
- CONCLUSION:
  - This trimodal approach was feasible, with an encouraging 26% 3-year survival rate.

- 6 year follow-up data.
  [Albain K, ASCO Meeting, 1999]
  - Plateau of 20% long-term survival, identical for both stage IIIA and stage IIIB disease.
  - CONCLUSIONS:
    - Response to induction chemotherapy plus XRT by computerized tomography (CT) scan is a poor predictor of outcome.
    - Clearance of mediastinal lymph node remains the strongest predictor of outcome for N_{2-3} disease.

- Intergroup 0139 Study.
  [Albain K, J Clin Oncol 23(16s): 624s (abstract 7014), 2005]
  - 396 eligible patients enrolled.
  - Stage IIIA (T_{1-3}, pN_2, M_0) NSCLC.
  - Patients were randomized to cisplatin/etoposide ×2 cycles with or without concurrent XRT (45 Gy).
  - Group I: surgery.
  - Group II: complete radiation to 61 Gy.
  - Then patients in both groups received another 2 cycles of cisplatin/etoposide.
  - RESULTS:
    - Group I: PFS is superior. Median survival 12.8 vs 10.5 months, $p = 0.017$, hazard ratio (HR) 0.77 (95% CI, 0.62–0.96). 5-year survival 22.4% vs 11.1%.
    - Median OS → 23.6 vs 22.2 months, $p = 0.24$, HR 0.87 (95% CI, 0.70–1.10). 5-year survival 27.2% vs 20.3%.

- – Longer follow-up in the Intergroup 0139 study confirms significantly improved PFS but not OS when surgery follows chemotherapy/XRT in patients with stage IIIA (pN_2) NSCLC.
  - – Trend for better 5-year OS with trimodal therapy.
  - – pN_0 at surgery predicts long-term survival.
- SIDE-EFFECTS:
  - – Treatment-related deaths:
    - – Group I: 16 (7.9%), of which 10 (5.0%) were within 30 days postoperatively.
    - – Group II: 4 (2.1%).
  - – Deaths by type of surgery:
    - – 5/23 (22%) simple and 9/31 (29%) complex pneumonectomies.
  - – 1/98 (1%) lobectomies.
- CONCLUSIONS:
  - – Surgery after chemotherapy/XRT can be considered in fit patients.
  - – This approach may not be optimal if a pneumonectomy is needed.

Superior sulcus tumors (Pancoast tumor)

- Historically therapy consisted of preoperative XRT followed by surgery.

- Some data suggest benefit for preoperative chemotherapy plus XRT followed by surgery.

- Induction chemotherapy plus XRT and surgical resection for NSCLC of the superior sulcus (SWOG 9416, Intergroup 0160).
  [Kraut MJ, *J Thorac Cardiovasc Surg* **121**(3): 472–483, 2001]
  - 111 patients with mediastinoscopy-negative $T_{3-4}N_{0-1}$ superior sulcus NSCLC.
  - Two cycles of cisplatin and etoposide chemotherapy concurrent with 45 Gy of XRT.
  - Patients with stable or responding disease underwent thoracotomy within 3–5 weeks.
  - All patients received two additional cycles of chemotherapy postoperatively.
  - RESULTS:
    - – 83/95 eligible patients underwent thoracotomy.
    - – 76 (92%) had a complete resection.
    - – The 2-year survival was 55% for all eligible patients, and 70% for patients who had a complete resection.

- SIDE-EFFECTS:
  - Cytopenia was the main grade 3 to 4 toxicity.
- CONCLUSION:
  - High complete response rates were achieved with resectability, and OS improved compared with historical experience, especially for T_4 tumors.

Adjuvant chemotherapy for non-small-cell lung cancer

[Mountain C, *Chest* **111**: 1710–1717, 1997]

- Outcomes with surgery alone are far from optimal.
  - Stage I ($T_1N_0M_0$) → 67% 5-year overall survival (OS) (10% local relapse, 15% distant).
  - Stage IIA ($T_1N_1M_0$) → 55% 5-year OS.
  - Stage IIIA ($T_xN_2M_0$) → 23% 5-year OS (15% local relapse, 60% distant relapse).

- Earlier trials (non-cisplatin-based therapy) failed to show a benefit for adjuvant chemotherapy

- Non-Small-Cell Lung Cancer Collaborative Group (NSCLCCG) meta-analysis.
  [NSCLCCG, *BMJ* **311**: 899–909, 1995]
  - Meta-analysis with individual patient data.
  - 9,387 patients in 52 chemotherapy trials in non-small-cell lung cancer (NSCLC).
  - Eight trials with 1,394 patients assessed postoperative cisplatin-based adjuvant chemotherapy.
  - RESULTS:
    - Hazard ratio (HR) 0.87 ($p = 0.08$), response rate 13%.
    - Absolute risk reduction 5% (95% CI, 1–10) in 5-year OS.
  - CONCLUSION:
    - This study rekindled interest in adjuvant chemotherapy in NSCLC.

- Italian Study.
  [Mineo T, *Eur J Cardiothorac Surg* **20**: 378–384, 2001]

- 66 patients with stage IB NSCLC were accrued over 7 years in this small, phase III trial of postoperative chemotherapy with six cycles of cisplatin 100 mg/m^2 on day 1 and etoposide 120 mg/m^2 on days 1–3, every 4 weeks, vs placebo.
- 3/4 of the patients received all six cycles of chemotherapy.
- RESULTS:
  - Median disease-free survival (DFS) was 77 months for the patients receiving chemotherapy vs 22 months for those who received placebo ($p = 0.02$).
  - The 5-year OS was 63% in the chemotherapy group and 45% in the placebo group ($p = 0.04$).

- IALT Trial (International Adjuvant Lung Cancer Trial).
  [Arriagada R, *New Engl J Med* **350**: 351–360, 2004]
  - 1,867 patients with stage I–III NSCLC were randomized within 60 days after surgical resection to receive observation alone or one of four different cisplatin-based regimens (80–120 mg/m^2 q 3–4 weeks).
    - Vindesine (3 mg/m^2 weekly ×5, then biweekly).
    - Vinblastine (4 mg/m^2 weekly ×5, then biweekly).
    - Vinorelbine (30 mg/m^2 weekly).
    - Etoposide (100 mg/m^2 on days 1–3 of each cycle).
  - Most commonly used regimen (49.3% of patients): cisplatin 100 mg/m^2 with etoposide for 3–4 cycles.
  - 27% of patients received postoperative radiation.
  - Median follow-up → 56 months.
  - RESULTS:
    - OS → 44.5% vs 40.4%, favoring the chemotherapy group with an HR of 0.86 (95% CI, 0.76–0.98) and $p < 0.03$.
  - SIDE EFFECTS:
    - Grade 3 or 4 toxicity was seen in 23% of patients in the treatment group.

- ALPI Trial (Adjuvant Lung Project Italy).
  [Scagliotti GC, *J Natl Cancer Inst* **95**: 1453–1461, 2004]
  - 1,209 patients with stage I to IIIA NSCLC within 42 days of surgical resection were randomized.
    - Group I: observation alone.
    - Group II: cisplatin 80 mg/m^2 on day 1 in combination with vindesine 3 mg/m^2 on days 1 and 8, every 28 days for 3 cycles.
  - 108 patients from one center were excluded from the analysis because of concerns about data integrity.

- 69% of patients in the treatment group completed the assigned chemotherapy.
- 43% of patients received postoperative radiation.
- Median follow-up → 64.5 months.
- RESULTS:
  - There were no statistically significant differences in median OS.
  - Median survival was 55 months in the chemotherapy group and 48 months in the observation group (HR 0.96; 95% CI, 0.81–1.13), $p = 0.589$).
- SIDE EFFECTS:
  - Grade 3 or 4 neutropenia was seen in 28% of patients in the treatment group.
  - Treatment-related mortality was seen in 7 patients in the observation group and 3 in the chemotherapy group.

- Japanese Oncology Group Trial 9304.
  [Otha M, *J Thorac Cardiovasc Surg* **106**: 703–706, 2003]
  - 119 patients with pathological N_2 disease were randomized within 6 weeks of surgery.
    - Group I: observation alone.
    - Group II: cisplatin 80 mg/m^2 on day 1 and vindesine 3 mg/m^2 on days 1 and 8, every 4 weeks for 3 cycles.
  - The trial was terminated early because of poor accrual.
  - 58% of treated patients received the target dose.
  - RESULTS:
    - Median survival → 36 months in both groups ($p = 0.89$).

- National Cancer Institute of Canada trial JBR.10 (NCI-CTG JBR.10).
  [Winton TL, *J Clin Oncol* **22**(Suppl): 621s (abstract 7018), 2004]
  - 482 patients with stage IB and II (except T_3N_0) NSCLC were randomized between treatment with four cycles of vinorelbine (initially 30 mg/m^2 weekly and then 25 mg/m^2 weekly because of toxicity) in combination with cisplatin (50 mg/m^2 on days 1 and 8 every 4 weeks) vs observation alone.
  - No postoperative radiation was administered.
  - Patients received 59% of the planned chemotherapy dose.
  - RESULTS:
    - Patients assigned chemotherapy had a significantly longer OS (94 vs 73 months, HR 0.69, $p = 0.0003$) and 5-year survival rates (69% vs 54%).
  - SIDE EFFECTS:
    - Febrile neutropenia was experienced by 7% of the patients who received chemotherapy.

- CALGB 9633 Trial (Cancer and Leukemia Group B).
  [Strauss GM, *J Clin Oncol* **22**(Suppl): 621s (abstract 7019), 2004]
  [Strauss GM, *Proc Am Soc Clin Oncol* **24**: abstract 7007, 2006]
  - 344 patients with stage IB ($T_2N_0M_0$) NSCLC were randomized:
    - Group I: observation alone.
    - Group II: carboplatin (AUC = 6) in combination with pacli-
      taxel (200 mg/m²) every 3 weeks for a total of 4 cycles.
  - 85% of planned chemotherapy doses were administered.
  - There was no planned postoperative radiation.
  - Median follow-up $\rightarrow$ 34 months.
  - RESULTS:
    - American Society of Clinical Oncology (ASCO) 2004 reported
      a statistically significant improvement in 4-year OS in the chemo-
      therapy group (71%; 95% CI, 0.62–0.81) vs the observation
      group (59%; 95% CI, 0.5–0.69).
  - SIDE EFFECTS:
    - 36% of patients in the chemotherapy group had grade 3 or 4
      neutropenia.
- These preliminary results were updated in ASCO 2006.
  - There was no longer a statistical significant difference in the median
    survival (95 vs 78 months, $p = 0.10$), or the 5-year survival of
    these two groups (59 vs 57 months, $p = 0.375$).
  - The only group that had a benefit in survival (by subset analysis)
    were patients with stage IB tumors > 4 cm diameter who statisti-
    cally survived longer if they received adjuvant chemotherapy
    (HR = 0.66; $p = 0.04$).

- ANITA Trial (Adjuvant Navelbine International Trialist Association).
  [Douillard JY, *Lancet Oncol* **7**(9): 719–727, 2006]
  - 840 patients with stage IB to IIIA NSCLC were randomized.
    - Group I: observation alone.
    - Group II: cisplatin 100 mg/m² every 4 weeks with vinorelbine
      30 mg/m² weekly for 16 weeks.
  - 76.1% of the planned doses were received.
  - Median follow-up > 70 months.
  - RESULTS:
    - Median survival $\rightarrow$ 65.8 months for the treatment group vs
      43.7 months for the observation group ($p = 0.0131$).
    - A subset analysis failed to demonstrate a benefit in patients
      with stage IB disease.
  - SIDE EFFECTS:
    - 12.5% of the patients had neutropenic fever.

- Uracil/Tegafur (UFT).
  [Hamada C, *J Clin Oncol* **22**(Suppl 14): A70, 2004]
  - UFT is not available in the USA.
  - Many trials have been conducted in Japan.
  - A 2,003 patient meta-analysis was presented at ASCO 2004.
  - RESULTS:
    - UFT significantly improved OS when compared with no chemotherapy (HR 0.74; 95% CI, 0.61–0.88).

In Summary

[The National Comprehensive Cancer Centers Practice Guidelines in Oncology v.2.2006 (http://www.nccn.org/professionals/physician_gls/PDF/nscl.pdf) reflects the actual consensus in the adjuvant therapy of NSCLC]

- Chemotherapy is indicated in patients with stage IB to III disease and in some patients with stage IA disease in the adjuvant treatment of resected NSCLC.

10

Combined modality therapy for locally advanced non-small-cell lung cancer

Radiation therapy for non-small-cell lung cancer

- Radiation Therapy Oncology Group (RTOG) 7301.
  [Perez C, *Cancer* **45**: 2744–2753, 1980]
  - Before 1980 the standard of care was radiation therapy (XRT) alone for this population, with survival rates of only 5% at 5 years.
  - Despite better local control there was no clear improvement in survival.

- Veterans Administration Surgical Adjuvant Group.
  [Higgins GA. Experience of the Veterans Administration Surgical Adjuvant Group. In: Muggia F, Rozencweig M (eds), *Lung Cancer: Progress in Therapeutic Research*. New York, Raven Press, 1979]
  - 246 patients with lung cancer (including small-cell lung cancer) were randomly assigned to receive supportive care only, and 308 received external-beam XRT to doses of 40–50 Gy.
  - The XRT was inadequate by modern standards, both in terms of the dose delivered (40–50 Gy) and the equipment used (orthovoltage).
  - XRT alone provided a modest but significant improvement in survival at 1 year (22% vs 16%, respectively).

- Role of XRT in combined modality treatment of locally advanced non-small-cell lung cancer (NSCLC).
  [Kubota K, *J Clin Oncol* **12**: 1547–1552, 1994]
  - Modest but significant improvement in 2-year survival rates in the range of 9–18%.

- 319 patients with locally advanced unresectable NSCLC were prospectively randomized.
  [Johnson DH, *Ann Intern Med* **113**: 33–38, 1990]
  - Group 1: chemotherapy alone with vindesine, 3 mg/m^2 twice weekly.
  - Group 2: standard thoracic XRT to a dose of 60 Gy over 6 weeks.
  - Group 3: combined vindesine and thoracic XRT.
  - RESULTS:
    - The overall response rate was superior in the XRT groups (XRT alone, 30%; XRT plus vindesine, 34%; vindesine alone, 10%; $p = 0.001$).
    - Median survival and overall survival (OS) were also comparable in all three groups.
  - LIMITATIONS OF THE STUDY:
    - A large number of patients in the vindesine-alone group received XRT.
    - The number of patients in the study was inadequate to detect a difference in survival.

Sequential chemotherapy followed by radiation therapy

- Sequential chemotherapy followed by XRT compared with XRT alone led to an improvement in median survival in two randomized trials.
  - Both trials involved cisplatin-based chemotherapy.
  - The standard of care evolved from XRT to chemotherapy followed by XRT.

- Cancer and Leukemia Group B (CALGB) 8433.
  [Dillman RO, *J Natl Cancer Inst* **88**: 1210–1215, 1996]
  [Dillman RO, *N Engl J Med* **323**: 940–945, 1990]
  - A randomized trial of induction chemotherapy plus high-dose XRT vs XRT alone in stage III NSCLC.
  - Used cisplatin (100 mg/m^2) days 1 and 29, and vinblastine (5 mg/m^2) weekly for two cycles, followed by XRT 60 Gy over 6 weeks, vs XRT alone.
  - RESULTS:
    - The study was terminated early, after accruing 78 patients in each group, due to a significant difference in median survival in favor of the sequential chemotherapy group (13.7 vs 9.6 months, $p = 0.01$).
    - 5-year survivals → 19% vs 7%.

- Randomized study with 353 patients with stage III NSCLC.
  [Le Chevalier T, *J Natl Cancer Inst* **83**: 417–423, 1991]
  - The standard group received XRT alone (65 Gy), and the other group received XRT plus chemotherapy (vindesine, cyclophosphamide, cisplatin, and lomustine).
  - RESULTS:
    - The 2-year survivals were 14% and 21% ($p = 0.08$) in the XRT alone and combined therapy groups, respectively.
    - The occurrence of distant metastasis was lower in the chemotherapy group ($p < 0.001$).

- There have also been randomized trials with negative results.
  [Trovo MG, *Cancer* **65**: 400–404, 1990]
  [Mattson K, *Eur J Cancer Clin Oncol* **24**: 477–482, 1988]
  [Morton RF, *Ann Intern Med* **115**: 681–686, 1991]
  [Mira JG, *Int J Radiat Oncol Biol Phys* **19**(Suppl): 145, 1990]
  - In two of the trials the treatment was cisplatin-based, with doxorubicin and cytoxan (CAP), and another two trials involved combinations of cyclophosphamide with less active agents such as methotrexate, procarbazine, and 5-fluorouracil.
  - LIMITATION OF THE STUDY:
    - These regimens are no longer used and are not considered to be as beneficial as the current platinum-based regimens.

- A meta-analysis in 1995 of the treatment of adjuvant and metastatic NSCLC showed that only platinum-based chemotherapy influences survival in NSCLC, and that the cyclophosphamide-based combinations may be detrimental to survival.
  [Non-Small Cell Lung Cancer Collaborating Group Metanalysis, *BMJ* **311**: 899–909, 1995]

- The results of the Cancer and Leukemia Group (CALG) 8433 study were later confirmed by an intergroup study (RTOG 8808, Eastern Cooperative Oncology Group (ECOG) 4588, Southwest Oncoogy Group (SWOG) 8992), and other clinical trials.
  [Sause WT, *J Natl Cancer Inst* **87**: 198–205, 1995]
  [Sause W, *Chest* **117**: 358–364, 2000]

- CALGB 9130
  [Clamon G, *J Clin Oncol* **17**: 4–11, 1999]
  - A randomized phase III study in patients with stage III NSCLC.
  - Randomized to cisplatin (100 mg/m^2 on days 1 and 29) + vinblastine (5 mg/m^2 weekly) followed by XRT, vs XRT alone, vs hyperfractionated XRT.

- RESULTS:
    - Median and 2-year survival in the chemoradiation group (13 months/31%) were superior to both standard XRT (11.4 months/20%) and hyperfractionated XRT (12.3 months/24%) (log rank, $p = 0.03$).

Concomitant administration of chemotherapy and radiotherapy for locally advanced disease

- Since several randomized studies, concurrent chemotherapy and XRT is now considered standard treatment in most cases of stage III disease. [American Society of Clinical Oncology. Clinical practice guidelines for the treatment of unresectable NSCLC. *J Clin Oncol* **22**(2): 330–353, 2004]

Concomitant chemoradiation: early trials

- Earlier studies were unable to prove benefit.
    - Combined modality therapy was not better, probably because of a lack of adequate chemotherapy and a lack of proper doses of XRT, and there was probably crossover.
- Southeastern Cancer Study Group(SECSG) study [Johnson DH, *Ann Intern Med* **113**: 33–38, 1990]
    - 319 patients with stage IIIA and IIIB disease were randomized to XRT alone (60 Gy over 6 weeks), vindesine alone (3 mg/m^2 weekly), or a combination of the two. Crossover was allowed.
    - RESULTS:
        - No differences in median survival were seen: 8.6 months, 10.1 months and 9.4 months ($p = 0.58$).
    - LIMITATIONS OF THE STUDY:
        - 5-year survival: 3%, 1% and 3%.
        - Vindesine is a drug with marginal activity in NSCLC.
- Three trials did not show benefit of using combination chemotherapy and XRT, vs XRT alone.
[Martini N, *Surg Clin North Am* **67**: 1037–1049, 1987]
[Soresi E, *Semin Oncol* **15**(Suppl 7): 20–25, 1987]
[Ansari R, *Proc Am Soc Clin Oncol* **10**: 241, 1991]
    - Martini used daily cisplatin (6 mg/m^2) and XRT (45 Gy).
    - Soresi used weekly cisplatin (15 mg/m^2).
    - Ansari used a more conventional every 3-weeks schedule (cisplatin 70 mg/m^2) with radiation doses of 50–60 Gy.

- The three studies were criticized because of the cisplatin schedules and doses used. In addition, the dose of radiation was low compared with the conventional current standard.

Concomitant chemoradiation: significant clinical trials

- European Organization for Research and Treatment of Cancer (EORTC) 08844.
  [Schaake-Koning C, *N Engl J Med* **326**: 524–530, 1992]
  - One of the first trials to show benefit.
  - 331 patients were randomized to receive daily cisplatin (6 mg/m^2) or weekly cisplatin (15 mg/m^2) with XRT, vs XRT alone.
  - Dose of radiation → 55 Gy.
  - RESULTS:
    - Survival in the daily cisplatin group was statistically significantly better compared with XRT alone (1-year survival, 54% vs 46%; 3-year survival, 16% vs 2%).
    - There was no significant difference between the weekly cisplatin group and the XRT-only group.

- The West Japan Group.
  [Furuse K, *J Clin Oncol* **17**(9): 2692–2699, 1999]
  - A phase III trial of concomitant chemoradiation, vs sequential chemotherapy followed by XRT.
  - 300 patients were treated.
  - Induction chemotherapy was mitomycin, cisplatin, and vindesine, and 56 Gy of daily XRT; concurrent chemoradiation was done with the same chemotherapy but split-course XRT.
  - RESULTS:
    - Concurrent treatment had a better median survival (16.5 vs 14.2 months) and better 5-year survival (16% vs 9%).

- RTOG 9410.
  [Curran WJ, *Proc Am Soc Clin Oncol* **22**: 621a (abstract 2499), 2003]
  - Designed to compare concomitant chemoradiation vs sequential chemotherapy and XRT.
  - A phase III randomized trial in unresectable stage III NSCLC.
  - Group 1 (sequential, standard, CALGB 8433): cisplatin and vinblastine followed by daily XRT to 60 Gy.
  - Group 2: chemotherapy with the same agents concomitantly with XRT.
  - Group 3: concurrent cisplatin and oral estoposide with hyperfractionated XRT (twice daily to a total dose of 69.6 Gy).

- RESULTS:
  - Concomitant chemoradiation was superior to sequential therapy (median survival 17 vs 14.6 months, $p = 0.038$).
  - Hyperfractionation was similar to conventional XRT.
  - Hyperfractionation gave better local control but more toxicity than conventional XRT.

- This randomized, phase II study was the third study to support the concomitant approach instead of the sequential one.
  [Zatloukal PV, *Lung Cancer* **46**: 87–98, 2004]
  - Chemotherapy in both groups consisted of 4 cycles of cisplatin 80 mg/m^2 on day 1 and vinorelbine 25 mg/m^2 on days 1, 8, and 15.
  - The dose of vinorelbine was ↓ to 12.5 mg/m^2 during cycles 2 and 3.
  - Cycles were repeated every 4 weeks.
  - In the concurrent group (group A) XRT was started from day 4 of cycle 2 (60 Gy/30 fractions/6 weeks).
  - In the sequential group (group B) XRT was started within 2 weeks of the completion of chemotherapy.
  - RESULTS:
    - The overall objective response rate was 80.4% (with 21.6% complete response (CR)) in group A and 46.8% (with 17% CR) in group B.
    - Median survival time in group A was 619 days and in group B 396 days ($p = 0.0216$, log rank test).
    - Median time to progression was 366 days in group A and 288 days in group B ($p = 0.0506$).
  - SIDE EFFECTS:
    - There was World Health Organization (WHO) grade 3 and 4 toxicity in groups A and B, respectively.
    - Anemia 11.8%, 6.3%; neutropenia 64.7%, 39.6%; thrombocytopenia 5.9%, 4.2%; esophagitis 17.6%, 4.2%, febrile neutropenia 7.8%, 2.1% of patients.

- NCP 95-01 Study (Groupe Français de Pneumo-Cancérologie).
  [Pierre F, *J Clin Oncol* **23**(25): 5910–5917, 2005]
  - 255 patients with locally advanced NSCLC were randomized in a phase III trial.
  - Sequential group: induction chemotherapy with cisplatin (120 mg/m^2) on days 1, 29, and 57, and vinorelbine (30 mg/m^2 weekly) from day 1 to day 78, followed by thoracic XRT at a dose of 66 Gy in 33 fractions.
  - Concurrent group: the same XRT was started on day 1 with two concurrent cycles of cisplatin 20 mg/m^2 daily and etoposide 50 mg/m^2

daily on days 1–5 and days 29–33; patients then received consolidation therapy with cisplatin 80 mg/m^2 on days 78 and 106 and vinorelbine 30 mg/m^2 weekly from day 78 to day 127.

- RESULTS:
  - Median survival was 14.5 months in the sequential group and 16.3 months in the concurrent group (log rank test, $p = 0.24$).
  - 2-, 3-, and 4-year survival rates were better in the concurrent group (39%, 25%, and 21%, respectively) than in the sequential group (26%, 19%, and 14%, respectively).
  - Esophageal toxicity was significantly more frequent in the concurrent group than in the sequential group (32% vs 3%).
- CONCLUSION:
  - Although not statistically significant, clinically important differences in the median, 2-, 3-, and 4-year survival rates were observed, with a trend in favor of concurrent chemoradiation therapy, suggesting that is the optimum strategy for patients with locally advanced NSCLC.

- In two meta-analyses of published data, the effect of the combined modality approach in patients with locally advanced disease resulted in a 12–24% ↓ in the risk of death at 1 year.
[Pritchard R, *Ann Intern Med* **125**: 723–729, 1996]
[Marino P, *Cancer* **76**: 593–601, 1995]

Induction or consolidation chemotherapy with concurrent chemoradiotherapy

- There have been efforts to integrate the concept of induction chemotherapy (before concurrent chemotherapy and XRT) or consolidation chemotherapy (after chemotherapy and XRT are finished) to improve response rate and survival.

- CALGB 9431.
[Vokes E, *J Clin Oncol* **20**(20): 4191–4198, 2002]
  - Explores the concept of chemotherapy followed by concomitant modality therapy.
  - Randomized, phase II study of cisplatin with gemcitabine or paclitaxel or vinorelbine as induction chemotherapy, followed by concomitant chemoradiotherapy for stage IIIB NSCLC.
  - Patients received four cycles of cisplatin 80 mg/m^2 on days 1, 22, 43, and 64 with:
    - Group 1: gemcitabine 1,250 mg/m^2 on days 1, 8, 22, and 29, and 600 mg/m^2 on days 43, 50, 64, and 71.

- Group 2: paclitaxel 225 mg/m^2 for 3 hours on days 1 and 22, and 135 mg/m^2 on days 43 and 64.
- Group 3: vinorelbine 25 mg/m^2 on days 1, 8, 15, 22, and 29, and 15 mg/m^2 on days 43, 50, 64, and 71.
- XRT was initiated on day 43 at 2 Gy/day (total dose 66 Gy).
- 175 eligible patients were analyzed.
- RESULTS:
  - Response rates after completion of XRT were 74%, 67%, and 73% for groups 1, 2, and 3, respectively.
  - Median survival for all patients was 17 months.
  - 1-, 2-, and 3-year survival rates were 68%/37%/28%, 62%/29%/19%, and 65%/40%/23% for the patients in groups 1, 2, and 3, respectively.
- CONCLUSION:
  - The observed survival rates exceed those of previous CALGB trials and may be attributable to the use of concomitant chemoradiotherapy.

- CALGB 39801.
  [Vokes EE, *Proc Am Soc Clin Oncol* **23**: 616 (abstract 7005), 2004]
  - 366 patients with stage III NSCLC were randomized.
    - Group 1 (182 patients): chemotherapy/XRT, carboplatin (AUC = 2) and paclitaxel (50 mg/m^2) each given weekly during 66 Gy chest XRT.
    - Group 2 (184 patients): two cycles of carboplatin (AUC = 6) and paclitaxel (200 mg/m^2) given q 21 days ×2 cycles followed by identical CT/XRT.
  - RESULTS:
    - Median survival in group 1 was 11.4 months vs 14 months in group 2 ($p = 0.154$).
    - 1-year survival estimates were 48% (41–57%) and 54% (47–62%) in groups 1 and 2, respectively.
    - The median survival achieved in each of the treatment groups is low compared to other recent experiences reported in the literature.
  - CONCLUSION:
    - The preliminary results from CALGB 39801 do not support the use of induction chemotherapy before definitive chemoradiotherapy.

- Other trials are including the concept of consolidation chemotherapy (as an alternative to induction chemotherapy) after combined modality therapy with the use of the same or other chemotherapy agents.

- SWOG 9019.
  [Albain KS, *J Clin Oncol* **20**: 3454–3460, 2002]
  - 50 patients with stage IIIB NSCLC in a phase II study.
  - Evaluated concurrent cisplatin (50 mg/m^2 on days 1, 8, 29, and 36) and etoposide (50 mg/m^2 on days 1–5 and 29–33) with 61 Gy XRT followed by consolidation chemotherapy, with cisplatin and etoposide for two more cycles.
  - RESULTS:
    - Median survival → 15 months.
    - 1-, 2-, 3-, and 5-year survivals were 58%, 34%, 17%, and 15%.
    - Superior to historic phase III sequential chemotherapy/XRT with 5-year survival rates of < 10%.

- SWOG 9504: consolidation docetaxel following concurrent chemoradiotherapy.
  [Gandara D, *Proc Am Soc Clin Oncol* **23**: 635 (abstract 7059), 2005]
  - Cisplatin (50 mg/m^2 on days 1, 8, 29, and 36), etoposide (50 mg/m^2 on days 1–5 and 29–33), and concurrent thoracic radiotherapy (total dose 61 Gy).
  - Consolidation docetaxel started 4–6 weeks after chemoradiotherapy at an initial dose of 75 mg/m^2.
  - 83 eligible patients: $T_4N_{0/1}$, 31 patients (37%); T_4N_2, 22 patients (27%); and $T_{1–3}N_3$, 30 patients (36%).
  - RESULTS:
    - Neutropenia during consolidation docetaxel was common (57% with grade 4).
    - Median progression-free survival (PFS) → 16 months.
    - Median survival → 26 months, and 1-, 2-, and 3-year survival rates were 76%, 54%, and 37%, respectively.
  - CONCLUSION:
    - Consolidation docetaxel results compared favorably with the preceding trial SWOG 9019, with better median and 1-, 2-, and 3-year survivals.

- Intergroup S0023 (SWOG 0023).
  [Kelly K, *Proc Am Soc Clin Oncol* **23**: 634s (abstract 7058), 2005]
  - Concurrent chemoradiotherapy followed by consolidation docetaxel and gefitinib (Iressa)/placebo maintenance.
  - Preliminary results of the phase III trial done to confirm the results of SWOG 9504.
  - 19-month median survival was higher than in most chemotherapy/XRT clinical trials for stage III disease.
  - Final results are eagerly awaited.

- Unfortunately, this trial showed that there is no role for maintenance gefinitib in NSCLC after chemotherapy and XRT.

- Randomized, phase II study of multimodality therapy in patients with stage III NSCLC.
  [Belani CP, *J Clin Oncol* **23**(25): 5883–5891, 2005]
  - Patients with unresected stage IIIA and IIIB NSCLC, received two cycles of induction paclitaxel (200 mg/m^2)/carboplatin (area under the plasma concentration time curve (AUC) = 6) followed by:
    - Group 1 (sequential): XRT (63.0 Gy).
    - Group 2 (induction/concurrent): two cycles of induction paclitaxel (200 mg/m^2)/carboplatin (AUC = 6) followed by weekly paclitaxel (45 mg/m^2)/carboplatin (AUC = 2) with concurrent XRT (63.0 Gy).
    - Group 3 (concurrent/consolidation): weekly paclitaxel (45 mg/m^2)/carboplatin (AUC = 2)/XRT (63.0 Gy) followed by two cycles of paclitaxel (200 mg/m^2)/carboplatin (AUC = 6).
  - RESULTS:
    - Median OS was 13.0, 12.7, and 16.3 months for groups 1, 2, and 3, respectively.
  - SIDE EFFECTS:
    - During induction chemotherapy, grade 3/4 granulocytopenia occurred in 32% and 38% of patients in groups 1 and 2, respectively.
    - The most common locoregional grade 3/4 toxicity during and after XRT was esophagitis, which was more pronounced with the administration of concurrent chemoradiotherapy in study groups 2 and 3 (19% and 28%, respectively).
  - CONCLUSION:
    - Concurrent weekly paclitaxel, carboplatin, and XRT followed by consolidation seems to be associated with the best outcome, although this schedule was associated with greater toxicity.

How to include surgery with combined modality therapy

- Evidence from recent trials, such as the North American Intergroup 0139 study, shows that multimodality therapy with surgery, XRT and chemotherapy might provide a superior outcome in locally advanced NSCLC.

- Neoadjuvant chemotherapy for NSCLC is discussed with more detail in Chapter 8.

- Two early trials with chemotherapy alone before surgery followed by surgery both showed an improvement in median survival (64 vs 11, and 26 vs 8 months) in favor of neoadjuvant chemotherapy followed by surgery instead of surgery alone.
  [Roth JA, *J Natl Cancer Inst* **86**: 673–680, 1994]
  [Rosell R, *N Engl J Med* **330**: 153–158, 1994]
  - The 3-year follow-up clearly established the advantage of chemotherapy before surgery compared with surgery alone, with median survivals of 56 vs 15 months in the Roth trial, and 23 vs 0 months in the Rosell trial.

- SWOG 8805.
  [Albain K, *Proc Am Soc Clin Oncol* **19**: 1888a, 2000]
  - 126 patients with stage III NSCLC were included, with 75 patients with N_2 (stage IIIA) and 51 patients with N_3 or T_4 (stage IIIB) disease.
  - Median follow-up → 6 years.
  - Patients received induction chemoradiation: two cycles of cisplatin/etoposide concomitantly with XRT (45 Gy).
  - Surgical resection was followed in case of clinical response (partial or complete) or stable disease.
  - RESULTS:
    - Overall response rate was 59%, plus 29% with stable disease.
    - Resectability was 85% for stage IIIA and 80% for stage IIIB.
    - There was no survival difference between the groups.
    - 3-year survival: 27% and 24%, stage IIIA and IIIB, respectively.
    - The strongest predictor of survival was mediastinal nodes present at surgery, with a median survival of 30 vs 10 months and a 3-year survival of 44% vs 18% ($p = 0.0005$).

- Intergroup 0139 (RTOG 9309).
  [Albain KS, *Proc Am Soc Clin Oncol* **23**(165 Part I/II) abstract 7014, 2005]
  - Phase III study of concurrent chemotherapy and XRT (chemo/XRT) vs chemo/XRT followed by surgical resection for stage IIIA (pN_2) NSCLC.
  - Surgery after chemo/XRT remains controversial for patients with stage IIIA (pN_2) NSCLC.
  - Initial analyses of Intergroup 0139 showed significantly better PFS, but no OS advantage, in the trimodality group.
  - With longer follow-up (≥ 2.5 years per patient), new analyses of the primary endpoints PFS and OS were conducted.

- 396 patients who had T_{1-3}, pN_2, M_0 NSCLC were enrolled (group 1, $n = 202$; group 2, $n = 194$).
- All patients received cisplatin (50 mg/m^2 on days 1, 8, 29, and 36), etoposide (50 mg/m^2 on days 1–5 and 29–33) (PE) and XRT (to 45 Gy starting day 1).
- Group 1: underwent resection if no progression (PD), and then PE ×2.
- Group 2: completed XRT to 61 Gy, with PE ×2.
- RESULTS:
  - Deaths: 5/23 (22%) simple and 9/31 (29%) complex pneumonectomies, 1/98 (1%) lobectomies.
  - Group 1: PFS is superior (median 12.8 vs 10.5 months, $p = 0.017$, hazard ratio (HR) 0.77; 5-year survival 22.4% vs 11.1%).
  - More patients in group 1 are alive without PD ($p = 0.008$), but more died without PD ($p = 0.021$).
  - OS curves overlap for 2 years, but separate later, favoring group 1 (median survival 23.6 vs 22.2 months, $p = 0.24$, HR = 0.8; 5-year survival 27.2% vs 20.3%; odds ratio for 5-year survival 0.63, $p = 0.10$).
  - Group 1: 5-year OS if pN_0 at surgery was 41%; if pN_{1-3} at surgery 24%; if no surgery 8% ($p < 0.0001$).
- CONCLUSIONS:
  - Longer follow-up of Intergroup 0139 confirms significantly improved PFS, but not OS when surgery follows chemo/XRT in patients with stage IIIA (pN_2) NSCLC.
  - There is a trend for better 5-year OS with trimodality therapy.
  - pN_0 at surgery predicts long-term survival.
  - Surgery after chemo/XRT can be considered in fit patients.
  - This approach may not be optimal if a pneumonectomy is needed.

Future directions in the treatment of locally advanced non-small-cell lung cancer

- From the 1980s to the 1990s to the present, the 5-year survival rates for patients with locally addvanced NSCLC have gradually improved, from approximately 5% with XRT alone, to 10% with sequential chemotherapy followed by XRT, to ~ 15% with concomitant chemoradiotherapy.

- The utility of consolidation chemotherapy needs to be verified in currently ongoing phase III clinical trials.

- The final doses and schedule of XRT might be improved.

- Published trials are suggesting the safe delivery of higher doses of XRT without increasing the rate of XRT pneumonitis.
  [ECOG 2597, Belani CP, J Clin Oncol 23: 3760–3767, 2005]
  [Socinski MA, Cancer 92: 1213–1223, 2001]
  [Socinski MA, J Clin Oncol 22: 4341–4350, 2004]

- The role of tyrosine kinase inhibitors (TKIs) and VEGF inhibitors, such as, bevacizumab in locally advanced NSLC is unclear at this point.
  - However, there is a lot of expectation that these inhibitors can be integrated in the multimodality therapy for locally advanced NSLC at some point (neoadjuvant therapy, adjuvant therapy, or concomitantly with XRT, etc.).
  - Several studies are ongoing.

11

Chemotherapy in advanced non-small-cell lung cancer

Prolongation of survival by chemotherapy

- Chemotherapy prolongs survival in advanced non-small-cell lung cancer (NSCLC).
  [Rapp E, *J Clin Oncol* **6**: 633–641, 1988]

- These reports showed an ↑ in survival in the patients receiving chemotherapy compared with those receiving best supportive care, and acceptable treatment costs.
  [Jaakkimainen L, *J Clin Oncol* **8**: 1301, 1990]

- Meta-analysis.
  [Souquet PJ, *Lancet* **342**: 19–21, 1993]
  [Marino P, *Chest* **106**: 861–865, 1994]
  [Marino P, *Cancer* **76**: 593–601, 1995]
  [Non-Small-Cell Collaborative Group, *Br Med J* **311**: 899–909, 1995]
  - All four meta-analyses support the same conclusion.
    - Chemotherapy prolongs survival time by a modest but statistically significant amount of time, and generally should be offered to patients.
    - Economic analyses support similar conclusions.
  - Alkylating agents were found to be detrimental.
  - Trials of cisplatin vs supportive care found a 27% ↓ in the risk of death and 10% improvement in survival in one year ($p < 0.0001$).

- [Spiro SG, *Thorax* **59**: 828–836, 2004]
  - 725 patients were randomized (364 chemotherapy, 361 no chemotherapy); 79% had WHO PS 0–1 stage disease.

- In addition to the primary treatment (surgery, radical radiotherapy, or best supportive care), patients were randomized to chemotherapy or no chemotherapy.
- Chemotherapy could be cisplatin + vindesine (CV), mitomycin + ifosfamide + cisplatin (MIC), mitomycin + vinblastine + cisplatin (MVP), or vinorelbine + cisplatin (NP).
- RESULTS:
  - There was significant survival advantage in the chemotherapy group: hazard ratio (HR) 0.77 (95% CI, 0.66–0.91), $p = 0.0015$.
- CONCLUSION:
  - The results confirm the previously reported overall survival benefit with cisplatin-based chemotherapy, as well as the improvement in median survival of ~8 weeks.
- SIDE-EFFECTS:
  - In the chemotherapy group, 28% had grade 3/4 toxicity, mainly hematological (12%), 4% had nausea/vomiting, 2% had neutropenic fever, and 14 (4%) reported treatment-related deaths.

Improvement in quality of life

- Chemotherapy improves quality of life (QOL) and symptoms in advanced NSCLC.
  [Ellis PA, *Br J Cancer* **71**: 366–370, 1995]
  - QOL scores improved with chemotherapy, whereas they declined over the first 6 weeks with best supportive care.
  - Symptomatic improvement was 70%, whereas the objective response rate (RR) was only 35%.
- ELVIS (Elderly Lung Cancer Vinorelbine Italian Study Group).
  [Elderly Lung Cancer Vinorelbine Italian Study Group, *J Natl Cancer Inst* **91**: 66–72, 1999]
  - Improved survival and QOL were demonstrated with single-agent chemotherapy in a population of patients aged > 70 years.
- Big Lung Trial (BLT).
  [Stephens RJ, *Proc Am Soc Clin Oncol* **21**: abstract 1161, 2002]
  [Spiro SG, *Thorax* **59**: 828–836, 2004]
  - QOL was assessed in a subgroup of 273 patients using patient-completed diary cards and the EORTC QLQ-C30 + LC17.
  - There was no evidence of a difference in the predefined primary QOL endpoint (global health status/QOL at 12 weeks) or in any of the secondary endpoints (physical functioning, emotional functioning, fatigue, pain, and dyspnea).

- Health service costs, estimated in a subgroup of 194 patients using retrospective resource use data collected from hospital records, showed no evidence of a significant offset between the cost of chemotherapy and the cost of symptom management.

Development of platin-based regimens

[Bunn PA, *Clin Cancer Res* **5**: 1087–1100, 1998]
[Johnson DH, *Clin Lung Cancer* **1**: 34–41, 1999]
[Vokes EE, *Chest* **106**: 659–661, 1994]

- Most traditional drugs have, at best, moderate single-agent activity in NSCLC.

- Complete responses to single-agent therapy are exceedingly rare.
  - Furthermore, the response duration is short, on average 2–3 months.
  - Median survival is 6–8 months, with no long-term survivors.

- Combination chemotherapy was investigated in an attempt to ↑ response rate.
  - Generally, higher responses were reported, but it remained unclear whether a more pronounced impact on survival was also achieved.

- CAMP (cytophosphamide, adriamycin, methotrexate, procarbazine) [Shepard KV, *Cancer* **56**: 2385–2390, 1985]

- One of the earliest combination chemotherapy regimens.
  - Single-institution study.
  - Response rate → 26%.

- Subsequent clinical trials incorporated cisplatin.

- Carboplatin and cisplatin are now considered to be the platform on which to build a regimen for NSCLC.
  - These drugs have a single-agent response rate of ~ 10% and different spectra of clinical toxicity.
    [Longeval E, *Cancer* **50**: 2751–2756, 1982]
    [Kris M, *Cancer Treat Rep* **70**: 1091–1096, 1986]
    [Eguchl K, *Eur J Cancer* **30A**: 188, 1994]
    [Shepherd FA, *Semin Oncol* **21** (Suppl 4): 48–62, 1994]

- The most frequently used combinations are regimens of cisplatin and etoposide, cisplatin and vinblastine, or (in Europe) cisplatin and vindesine or teniposide.
  - Phase II studies of these regimens resulted in a response rate →

30–50%, suggesting higher activity than for the first-generation combination regimens.
[Jett JR, *Mayo Clin Proc* **68**: 603–661, 1993]

- Direct comparisons of cisplatin-based regimens with non-cisplatin-containing combinations have been performed.
  - Three studies reported superior survival with cisplatin.

- Southwest Oncology Group (SWOG) 8738.
  [Gandara DR, *J Clin Oncol* **11**(5): 873–878, 1993]
  - A phase III study.
  - Dose–response curve for cisplatin activity in NSCLC.
  - Doses of 100–200 mg/m^2 have <u>not</u> improved survival.

- Eastern Cooperative Oncology Group (ECOG) 1581.
  [Bonomi P, *J Clin Oncol* **7**: 1602–1613, 1989]
  - CAMP vs three cisplatin-containing regimens, including the combination of mitomycin C, vinblastine, and cisplatin (MVP).
  - MVP produced the highest numeric response rate → 31%; median survival time → 4.5 (for MVP) to 6.5 months and was not significantly different among the four regimens.
  - Carboplatin or iproplatin followed by MVP chemotherapy at the time of first progression was compared with first-line MVP and two other cisplatin-based regimens.
  - Patients treated with initial carboplatin had the longest median survival time.
  - First-line MVP again resulted in the highest response rate, but in a lower median survival time (23 vs 32 weeks for initial carboplatin).

Development of third-generation chemotherapy agents in the 1990s

- Randomized studies in the 1980s established the combination of cisplatin with etoposide or vinblastine as a standard therapy.
  - During the last decade several new agents emerged as treatment options, as single agents or in combinations.

Vinorelbine

- European multicenter trial.
  [Le Chevalier T, *J Clin Oncol* **12**: 360–367, 1994]
  - 612 patients.

- RESULTS:
  - Median survival time → 30 weeks for patients treated with cisplatin and vindesine.
  - Patients treated with cisplatin and vinorelbine had a significantly longer median survival time → 40 weeks.
- Vinorelbine vs vinorelbine plus cisplatin in advanced NSCLC. [Depierre A, *Ann Oncol* **5**: 37–42, 1994]
  - Randomized trial.
  - Combination of cisplatin plus vinorelbine proved superior to the single agent.
- ELVIS (Elderly Lung Cancer Vinorelbine Italian Study Group). [Elderly Lung Cancer Vinorelbine Italian Study Group, *J Natl Cancer Inst* **91**: 66–72, 1999]
  - Effects of vinorelbine on QOL and survival of elderly patients with advanced NSCLC.
  - Vinorelbine was best supportive care in the elderly (age ≥ 70 years).
  - ↑ median survival (6.5 vs 4.9 months) and QOL.

Paclitaxel

- ECOG 5592.
  [Bonomi P, *Proc Am Soc Clin Oncol* **15**: 382 (abstract 1145), 1996]
  - Three-arm, phase III trial comparing etoposide + cisplatin vs paclitaxel with cisplatin + G-CSF (G) vs paclitaxel + cisplatin in advanced NSCLC.
  - RESULTS:
    - Paclitaxel (24-hour infusion) + cisplatin was superior to the etoposide + cisplatin regimen.
    - No evidence of ↑ response rate with higher paclitaxel dose.
- [Giaccone G, *J Clin Oncol* **16**(6): 2133–2141, 1998]
  - Randomized study of paclitaxel + cisplatin vs cisplatin + teniposide in patients with advanced NSCLC.
  - Cisplatin + paclitaxel resulted in a median survival (10 months) similar to that with cisplatin + teniposide, but was better tolerated.
- [Belani C, *Proc Am Soc Clin Oncol* **17**: 455a (abstract 1751), 1998]
  - Randomized, phase III trial cisplatin + etoposide vs carboplatin + paclitaxel in advanced and metastatic NSCLC.
  - RESULTS:
    - Identical median survival times → 8 months.

- SIDE-EFFECTS:
  - ↑ nausea, vomiting, and myelosuppression with cisplatin.
  - ↑ neurotoxicity with carboplatin.

Gemcitabine

- Cisplatin ± gemcitabine in patients with advanced NSCLC.
  [Sandler A, *Proc Am Soc Clin Oncol* 17: 454a (abstract 1747), 1998]
  - Phase III study.
  - RESULTS:
    - Combination of gemcitabine + cisplatin showed a significant improvement in median survival (7.6 vs 9.1 months) vs single-agent cisplatin.

- Gemcitabine + cisplatin vs etoposide + cisplatin in the treatment of locally advanced or metastatic NSCLC.
  [Cardenal F, *J Clin Oncol* 17: 12–18, 1999]
  - Randomized, phase III study.
  - RESULTS:
    - Suggested a favorable impact on median survival for gemcitabine + cisplatin.

Docetaxel

- The Japanese Taxotere Lung Cancer Study Group.
  [Kubota K, *J Clin Oncol* 22(2): 254–261, 2004]
  [Kunitoh H, *Proc Am Soc Clin Oncol* 20: 323a (abstract 1289), 2001]
  - Phase III, randomized trial.
  - 151 patients per group.
  - Dose:
    - Docetaxel (Taxotere) (60 mg/m^2 1-hour i.v.) + cisplatin (80 mg/m^2 2-hour i.v., q 3–4 weeks) ×2 cycles.
    - Vindesine (3 mg/m^2 i.v. bolus on days 1, 8, and 15) + cisplatin (80 mg/m^2 2-hour i.v. on day 1, q 3–4 weeks) ×2 cycles.
  - RESULTS:
    - Docetaxel/cisplatin overall response rate (ORR) → 37% vs 21%, $p < 0.01$.
    - Median survival → 11.3 vs 9.6 months.
    - 2-year survival → 24% vs 12%.
  - CONCLUSION:
    - Docetaxel/cisplatin gave a better ORR, median survival, and 2-year survival.

Combination chemotherapy with third-generation agents is better than single agents alone

- Several randomized studies have proven that the combination of third-generation chemotherapeutic agents in doublets gives superior response and survival than single-agent chemotherapy.

- CALGB 9730.
  [Lilenbaum RC, *J Clin Oncol* **23**(1): 190–196, 2005]
  - Phase III, randomized trial of carboplatin + paclitaxel vs paclitaxel alone in patients with stage IIIB (malignant effusion) and stage IV disease.
  - Paclitaxel 225 mg/m^2 over 3 hours or the same; carboplatin + paclitaxel at AUC of 6, both i.v. on day 1 every 3 weeks for up to 6 cycles.
  - 584 patients were entered in study.
  - RESULTS:
    - Response rate → paclitaxel 16% and carboplatin + paclitaxel 30% ($p < 0.0001$).
    - Survival distributions were significantly different in favor of carboplatin + paclitaxel ($p = 0.023$).
    - Median survival → 6.5 months for paclitaxel and 8.5 months for carboplatin + paclitaxel.
    - 1-year survival rates → 31% for paclitaxel and 36% for carboplatin + paclitaxel ($p = $ NS).
  - SIDE-EFFECTS:
    - Grade 3/4 toxicities (% paclitaxel/carboplatin + paclitaxel): absolute neutrophil count (ANC) 32/62, febrile neutropenia 5/8, platelets 1/11, hemoglobin 3/13, nausea/vomiting 4/9, peripheral neuropathy 13/15. Any grade 3–4 toxicity (%): 71/89 ($p < 0.0001$).

- Swedish Lung Cancer Study Group.
  [Sederholm C, *Semin Oncol* **29**(3 Suppl 9): 50–54, 2002]
  - Phase III study; 332 patients with advanced NSCLC were randomized to gemcitabine (G) or gemcitabine + carboplatin (G + C).
  - Dose:
    - G: 1,250 mg/m^2 i.v. on days 1 and 8, q 21 days.
    - G + C: same regimen of G, with C at AUC = 5, i.v. on day 1, q 21 days.
  - RESULTS:
    - Objective response rate for the first 275 patients assessed.
    - 12% for G (complete response/partial response (CR/PR) = 0/12%) and 30% for G + C (CR/PR = 2/28%).

- Time to progression for G/G + C → 4/6 months (p = 0.001).
  - Median survival for all patients → 9 months.
- SIDE-EFFECTS:
  - Hematologic toxicities for G were all less than WHO grade 2. For G + C, grade 3/4 toxicities (% of cycles) were: anemia 1.5/0.1, leukopenia 12.6/0.4, and thrombocytopenia 15.2/8.9.

- Docetaxel vs docetaxel + cisplatin in patients with advanced NSCLC. [Georgoulias V, *Clin Lung Cancer* **4**(5): 288–293, 2003]
  - Preliminary analysis of a multicenter, randomized, phase III study.
  - 307 chemotherapy-naive patients were treated:
    - Group A (n = 149): docetaxel (100 mg/m^2 on day 1).
    - Group B (n = 158): docetaxel (100 mg/m^2 on day 1) + cisplatin (80 mg/m^2 on day 2) and rhG-CSF (5 μg/kgr s.c. on days 3–8).
  - Cycles were repeated every 3 weeks.
  - RESULTS:
    - ORR was 18% vs 35% in groups A and B, respectively (p < 0.001).
    - Stable disease (SD) → 22% vs 22%.
    - Median survival: 10 vs 13 months.
  - SIDE-EFFECTS:
    - Grade 3/4 toxicities (WHO criteria) in groups A/B were: neutropenia 30 (21%)/39 (25%); nausea/vomiting 0 (0%)/7 (4%); grade 2–4 asthenia 28 (19%)/36 (27%).
    - There were five treatment-related deaths in group B.

The best chemotherapeutic combination with third-generation agents for non-small-cell lung cancer

- The consensus is that most of the chemotherapy combinations with these agents are equivalent, and the choice for a particular patient's treatment is probably based in the toxicity profile of the combinations.

- ECOG 1594.
  [Schiller JH, *N Engl J Med* **346**: 92–98, 2002]
  - One of the first studies to introduce the carboplatin + paclitaxel combination, it established the similarity between all the drug combinations.
  - ~ 290 patients per group.
  - Dose:
    - Group A: paclitaxel (Taxol) 135 mg/m^2 over 24 hours on day 1, and cisplatin 75 mg/m^2 on day 2.

- – Group B: gemcitabine 1000 mg/m^2 on days 1, 8, and 15, and cisplatin 100 mg/m^2 on day 1.
- – Group C: docetaxel (Taxotere) 75 mg/m^2 on day 1 and cisplatin 75 mg/m^2 on day 1.
- – Group D: paclitaxel (Taxol) 225 mg/m^2 over 3 hours on day 1, and carboplatin (AUC = 6) on day 1.
- RESULTS:
  - – CR: ≤ 1% in all groups.

	Group				p
	A	B	C	D	
Overall RR (%) →	21.3	21	17.4	15.3	A vs D: 0.075
TTP (months) →	3.5	4.5	3.6	3.3	B vs A: 0.003
Median survival → (months)	7.9	8.1	7.4	8.3	
1-year survival (%) →	31	36	31	34	

- SWOG 9509.
  [Kelly K, *J Clin Oncol* **19**: 3210–3218, 2001]
  - Confirmed the similar efficacy of platinum combinations, and consolidated the role of paclitaxel + carboplatin as the standard regimen and future reference for cooperative studies.
  - Phase III, randomized trial compared efficacy as well as toxicity, tolerability, QOL, and resource utilization between vinorelbine + cisplatin and paclitaxel + carboplatin.
  - RESULTS:
    - – ORR and 1-year survival rates → 28% and 25%, and 36% and 38%, respectively.
    - – Median survival → 8 months in both groups.
  - SIDE-EFFECTS:
    - – More grade 3/4 myelosuppression (leukopenia and neutropenia) and grade 3 nausea and vomiting in the vinorelbine + cisplatin group.
    - – Higher grade 3 peripheral neuropathy in the paclitaxel + carboplatin group.
  - CONCLUSION:
    - – No difference in QOL was observed, and the overall costs in the paclitaxel + carboplatin group were higher, mainly because of drug costs.

- TAX326.
  [Fossella F, *J Clin Oncol* **21**: 3016–3024, 2003]
  - One of the largest randomized, phase III studies, which suggested superiority of the cisplatin + docetaxel combination and similarity of the carboplatin + docetaxel combination compared with cisplatin + vinorelbine.
  - Docetaxel (Taxotere)/cisplatin (TC) and docetaxel/carboplatin (TCb) vs vinorelbine/cisplatin (VC), ~ 400 patients per group.
  - RESULTS:

	TC	TCb	VC	*p*
Median survival (months)	10.9	9.1	10	TC vs VC: 0.046
1-year survival (%)	47	38	42	
2-year survival (%)	21	17	14	TC vs VC: 0.035

  - SIDE-EFFECTS:

	TC	TCb	VC	*p*
Grade 3/4 anemia (%)	7	10	24	TC and TCb vs VC: < 0.01
Grade 3/4 neutropenia (%)	75	74	79	
Nausea (%)	10	6	16	TC and TCb vs VC: < 0.01
Vomiting (%)	8	4	16	TC and TCb vs VC: < 0.01
Weight loss > 10% (%)	7	7	15	TC and TCb vs VC: < 0.01

- EORTC 08975.
  [Smit EF, *J Clin Oncol* **21**: 3909–3917, 2003]
  - Randomized, phase III trial of three chemotherapy regimens in advanced NSCLC.
  - 160 patients per group.
  - Equivalent survival between the platinum groups, but inferior results in the paclitaxel + gemcitabine group.

- RESULTS:

	Pac + Cis	Gem + Cis	Pac + Gem
Response rate (%)	31.0	36.0	27
Progression-free survival (months)	4.4	5.6 ($p = 0.03$)	3.9 ($p = 0.08$)
Median survival time (months)	8.1	8.8 ($p = 0.9$)	6.9 ($p = 0.091$)
1-year survival (%)	36	33	27

Cis, cisplatin; Gem, gemcitabine (Gemzar).

- Italian Lung Cancer Project Study.
  [Scagliotti GV, *J Clin Oncol* **20**: 4285–4291, 2002]
  - Phase III, randomized trial comparing three platinum-based doublets in advanced NSCLC.
  - Cisplatin + gemcitabine, carboplatin + paclitaxel, cisplatin + vinorelbine.
  - 200 patients per group.
  - RESULTS:

	Cis + Gem	Car + Pac	Cis + Vin
Median survival (months)	9.8	9.9	9.5
Response rate (%)	30	32	31
1-year survival (%)	37	43	37

  - Identical median survival, response rate, and 1-year survival.
  - SIDE-EFFECTS:
    - Neutropenia was significantly higher with vinorelbine (43% vs 35% vs 17% of cycles, $p < 0.001$).
    - Thrombocytopenia with gemcitabine (16% of cycles, $p < 0.001$).
    - Alopecia and peripheral neurotoxicity were most common with paclitaxel.

- The Four-Arm Cooperative Study (FACS) (Japan).
  [Kubota K, *Proc Am Soc Clin Oncol* **22**: 618s (abstract 7006), 2004]
  - This randomized, phase III trial included irinotecan + cisplatin as the Japanese reference regimen, and allowed the first direct comparison of this regimen with other widely tested platinum doublets.
  - The FACS compared three platinum-based combinations, gemcitabine + cispaltin, vinorelbine + cisplatin, and paclitaxel + carbo-

platin, with cisplatin + irinotecan as the reference group.
- Chemotherapy-naive patients with stage IIIB or IV NSCLC.
- 602 patients were registered from 44 hospitals in Japan.
- RESULTS:
  - Because no inferiority of any of the three experimental regimens was demonstrated, irinotecan + cisplatin remains the standard regimen and future reference in Japan.
  - The 1-year survival rate of 59.2% in the reference group was higher than expected.
- SIDE-EFFECTS:
  - Toxicities were dependent on the regimen being used.
  - More thrombocytopenia with gemcitabine.
  - More neuropathy with paclitaxel.
  - More diarrhea with irinotecan.
  - More nausea/vomiting with cisplatin.

	Pac + Car	Gem + Cis	Nav + Cis	Iri + Cis
No. of patients (efficacy)	145	146	145	145
1-year survival (%)	51.0	59.6	48.3	59.2
Median survival time (months)	12.3	14.8	11.4	14.2
Response rate (%)	32.4	30.1	33.1	31.0

Non-platin combinations in non-small-cell lung cancer

- Coalition Study (USA): Alpha Oncology Trial (A1–99002L).
  [Treat J, *Proc Am Soc Clin Oncol* **23**: 627s (abstract 7025), 2005]
  - In the USA, the Coalition of National Cancer Cooperative Groups reported similar results in a study where the three groups in question above were compared directly.
  - Using paclitaxel + carboplatin as the reference regimen, this study randomized patients to two additional groups: paclitaxel + gemcitabine and gemcitabine + carboplatin.
  - 929 chemotherapy-naive patients, including those with treated brain metastasis, were enrolled.
  - The primary endpoint was overall survival, with time to progression (response rate) and QOL evaluation as secondary endpoints.

- RESULTS:

	Overall	Gem + Carb	Gem + Pac	Pac + Carb
ORR (%)	39.5	33.6	43.6	41.6
Median survival time (months)	7.7	7.6	8.4	7.9
1-year survival (%)	33	31	33	33
2-year survival (%)	10	8	8	11

- SIDE-EFFECTS:
  - The incidence and grade of toxicity with the three regimens were comparable.
  - Anemia and thrombocytopenia were more common with gemcitabine + carboplatin.
  - Alopecia and neuropathy were more common in the paclitaxel-containing regimens.

- Paclitaxel + carboplatin (PC) vs paclitaxel + gemcitabine (PG) in advanced NSCLC.
  [Kosmidis P, J Clin Oncol 20: 3578–3585, 2002]
  - Phase III, randomized trial.
  - 509 patients, PS 0–2 disease.
  - Inoperable, recurrent or metastatic NSCLC.
  - PC: paclitaxel 200 mg/m^2 and carboplatin AUC = 6 on day 1.
  - PG: paclitaxel 200 mg/m^2 on day 1, gemcitabine 1,000 mg/m^2 on days 1 and 8.
  - RESULTS:
    - ORR: 28% (PC) vs 35% (PG).
    - Median survival: PC 10.4 months vs PG 9.8 months.
    - 1-year survival: 41.7% (PC) vs 41.4% (PG).
    - 2-year survival: 17% (PC) vs 15.2% (PG).
    - Patients with PS 0–1 vs PS 2 had a median survival of 11.1 vs 5.9 months ($p < 0.05$).
  - SIDE-EFFECTS:
    - Grade 3/4 neutropenia: 15% both groups.
    - Grade 3/4 thrombocytopenia.

- ACORN 9901 (American Clinical Oncology Research Network Randomized Multicenter Study).
  [Bosserman L, Proc Am Soc Clin Oncol 20: 279b (abstract 2868), 2001]

- Weekly docetaxel (Taxotere) + gemcitabine vs weekly paclitaxel + gemcitabine in advanced NSCLC.
  - Docetaxel 40 mg/m^2 i.v. on days 1 and 8 + gemcitabine 1,200 mg/m^2 i.v. on days 1 and 8.
  - Repeat q 3 weeks (27 patients).
  - Paclitaxel 120 mg/m^2 i.v. on days 1 and 8 + gemcitabine 1,200 mg/m^2 i.v. on days 1 and 8.
  - Repeat q 3 weeks (30 patients).
  - RESULTS:
    - PR 44% vs 37% in favor of docetaxel.

- Vinorelbine + cisplatin vs docetaxel + gemcitabine in advanced NSCLC.
  [Georgoulias V, *J Clin Oncol* **23**: 2937–2945, 2005]
  - Phase III, randomized trial, 251 chemotherapy-naive patients.
  - Dose:
    - Group A: docetaxel (100 mg/m^2 on day 8) and gemcitabine (1,000 mg/m^2 on days 1 and 8) or
    - Group B: vinorelbine (30 mg/m^2 on days 1 and 8) and cisplatin (80 mg/m^2 on day 8).
    - rhG-CSF (150 μg/m^2 s.c.) was given to all patients (days 9–15).
  - RESULTS:
    - ORR → 29% vs 36%.
    - SD: 23% vs 19%.
    - Median survival → 9 vs 11.5 months
  - SIDE-EFFECTS:
    - Toxicity by WHO criteria (group A/B) was: grade 3/4 neutropenia 23 (17%)/37 (32%) ($p = 0.007$); grade 3 fatigue 9 (7%)/16 (14%) ($p = 0.066$); 3 toxic deaths occurred in group B.

- Gemcitabine + vinorelbine compared with cisplatin + vinorelbine or cisplatin + gemcitabine for advanced NSCLC.
  [Gridelli C, *J Clin Oncol* **21**: 3025–3034, 2003]
  - Italian GEMVIN Investigators and the National Cancer Institute of Canada Clinical Trials Group.
  - Phase III trial comparing gemcitabine + vinorelbine (GV) with cis/vinorelbine + cis/gemcitabine (PCT) for advanced NSCLC.
  - 501 patients, of which 415 were evaluable for QOL analysis.
  - RESULTS:
    - Median OS: 38 (PCT) vs 32 (GV) weeks (one-sided, $p = 0.08$).
    - Median PFS: 22 (PCT) vs 17 (GV) weeks (one-sided, $p = 0.005$).
    - ORR: 29% (PCT) vs 26% (GV) (two-sided, $p = 0.38$).

- GV is associated with less severe gastrointestinal, hematologic, and auditory toxicity compared with PCT.
- GV patients are less likely to have worsening of QOL.
- There was no significant difference in OS.
- PCT has a significantly longer PFS and a trend to improvement in some disease-related symptoms.
- SIDE-EFFECTS:
  - There was no significant difference in general QOL or functional scales; PCT patients had improved disease-related symptoms (not significant on multivariable analysis), and worsening appetite, vomiting and alopecia (significant).
  - PCT patients had significantly more grade 3/4 neutropenia, vomiting, alopecia, and ototoxicity.
- Paclitaxel + gemcitabine (PG) vs gemcitabine + carboplatin (GC). [Kosmidis P, *Proc Am Soc Clin Oncol* **23**(16s): abstract 7000, 2005]
  - A multicenter, phase III, randomized trial in patients with advanced inoperable NSCLC.
  - 512 patients randomized, stage IIIB/IV, ECOG PS 0 and 1.
  - RESULTS:
    - Median survival: 10 and 10.5 months (PG vs GC).
    - 1-year survival: 44% vs 42% (PG vs GC).
  - SIDE-EFFECTS:
    - Hematologic toxicites worse with GC.
    - Alopecia and neurotoxicity worse with PG.

Combination chemotherapy using 'triplets' (three agents)

- Different combinations have been attempted in several clinical trials.
  - None of them have shown a significant ↑ in response rate without ↑ the toxicity profile.
  - There is no recommendation for the use of triplets in NSCLC.

Combination chemotherapy with targeted agents

- > 10 randomized studies unsuccessfully tried to ↑ the response.
  - Among the agents used were: protein kinase C (ISIS 3521), farnesyltransferase inhibitors (FTIs), matrix metalloproteinase (MMPs; e.g. AG3340 and BMS275291), epidermal growth factor receptor (EGFR) tyrosine kinase inhibitors (gefitinib and erlotinib), and an FTI (ras) (lonafarnib).

– We describe here three of the studies reported in ASCO 2005; this topic is discussed further in Chapter 18.

• Two randomized, phase III studies of bexarotene were presented at ASCO 2005.
  [Blumenschein R, *Proc Am Soc Clin Oncol* **23**: 621 (abstract 7001), 2005]
  [Jassem J, *Proc Am Soc Clin Oncol* **23**: 627 (abstract 7024), 2005]
  • Carboplatin + paclitaxel ± bexarotene, or cisplatin + vinorelbine ± bexarotene.
  • RESULTS:
    – No improvement in survival was seen with the addition of bexarotene to chemotherapy.
    – Hyperlipidemia correlated with response to therapy.

• Randomized, phase III trial in PS 2 patients only; carboplatin + paclitaxel vs carboplatin + paclitaxel poliglumex (PPX).
  [Langer C, Proc Am Soc Clin Oncol **23**: 623s (abstract 7011), 2005]
  • RESULTS:
    – No difference in survival with the use of PPX.
    – Advantages of PPX: administration time, no need for premedication, no alopecia.

Best combination chemotherapy

• ECOG 4599.
  [Sandler A, *Proc Am Soc Clin Oncol* **23**: abstract LBA4 and oral presentation, 2005]
  • 850 patients were randomized in a phase III trial for first-line treatment of NSCLC.
  • Carboplatin (AUC = 6) + paclitaxel (200 mg/m^2) ± bevacizumab (15 mg/kg).
  • Inclusion criteria:
    – Chemotherapy-naive, stage IIIB (pleural or pericardial effusion only) or stage IV non-squamous NSCLC.
    – Measurable or non-measurable disease.
    – ECOG PS 0–1.
    – International normalized ratio (INR) < 1.5 and a prothrombin time no greater than upper limits of normal within 1 week prior to randomization.
    – No history of thrombotic or hemorrhagic disorders.
    – No gross hemoptysis (defined as bright-red blood of a ½ teaspoon or more).

- Brain metastases were NOT allowed.
- RESULTS:
  - Significant prolongation of PFS at 1 year from 6.4% to 14.6%, and 1-year survival from 43.7% → 51.9%.
  - Median survival ↑ from 10.2 → 12.5 months.
  - Median PFS ↑ from 4.5 → 6.4 months.
- SIDE-EFFECTS:
  - Pulmonary hemorrhage in carboplatin + paclitaxel ± bevacizumab group 1.2% vs 0% in carboplatin + paclitaxel group.
  - 8 patients died from treatment complications, and 5 of these 8 died from bleeding complications, resulting in 4.5% mortality rate vs 1% for controls (history of hemoptysis, squamous cell histology, and brain metastatic disease).
- CONCLUSION:
  - This study of combination chemotherapy with carboplatin + paclitaxel ± bevacizumab in the treatment of NSCLC is a landmark study because it is the first to show that a targeted agent can ↑ survival and time to progression.

New chemotherapy agents for non-small-cell lung cancer

Bortezomib (Velcade)

- Bortezomib ± docetaxel in previously treated patients with advanced NSCLC.
  [Fanucchi M, *J Clin Oncol* **22**(Suppl 14s): 643s (abstract 7034), 2004]
  [Fanucchi M, *Lung Cancer* **49**(Suppl 2): S30 (abstract), 2005]
  - Bortezomib is a reversible inhibitor of the chymotrypsin-like activity of the 26S proteasome in mammalian cells.
    - The 26S proteasome is a large protein complex that degrades ubiquitinated proteins.
    - The ubiquitin–proteasome pathway plays an essential role in regulating the intracellular concentration of specific proteins, thereby maintaining homeostasis within cells.
    - Inhibition of the 26S proteasome prevents this targeted proteolysis, which can affect multiple signaling cascades within the cell.
  - A randomized, phase II study of bortezomib + docetaxel vs bortezomib alone for stage IIIB or IV NSCLC, and one prior chemotherapy regimen was reported.
    - Group A: bortezomib 1.5 mg/m^2 i.v. bolus.

- Group B: docetaxel 75 mg/m^2 i.v. + bortezomib 1.3 mg/m^2.
- RESULTS:
  - Group A → PR rate → 10.0% vs 15.6% in group B.
  - Median time to progression → 42.5 days in group A and 86 days in group B.
  - Median duration of response → 9.8 months in group A; has not yet been reached in group B.
- SIDE-EFFECTS:
  - The most common ≥ grade 3 events were dehydration, nausea, and vomiting in group A, and neutropenia, fatigue, and diarrhea in group B.
- CONCLUSION:
  - Phase III trials are eagerly awaited to confirm the utility of bortezomib in NSCLC.

Telcyta (TLK286)

- A glutathione analog prodrug.

- TLK286 is the first in a new class of investigational cancer-cell-activated chemotherapeutic agents.

- It was designed to exploit the overexpression of glutathione S-transferase P1-1 (GST P1-1), an enzyme that is overexpressed in many human cancer cells.

- High levels of GST P1-1 are associated with a poor prognosis and resistance to certain chemotherapeutic agents.

- Preclinical studies suggest that activation of TLK286 occurs when GST P1-1 splits TLK286 into two active fragments: a glutathione analog fragment and an active cytotoxic fragment.
  - The cytotoxic fragment reacts with important cell components, including RNA, DNA and proteins, leading to cell death.
  - The results suggest that TLK286 is synergistic when combined with some chemotherapeutic drugs, including platinum compounds, taxanes, and anthracyclines.

- A phase I/II study with planned doses of TLK286 of 400, 500, 750, or 1000 mg/m^2 combined with standard doses of carboplatin (AUC = 6) and paclitaxel (200 mg/m^2) i.v. q 3 weeks.
  [Sequist LV, *Proc Am Soc Clin Oncol* **23**: abstract 7275, 2005]
  - Interim analysis → no dose-limiting toxicities (DLTs) have been observed.

- 2 patients had grade 3/4 neutropenia, which resolved before the next treatment cycle.
- No febrile neutropenia was seen. Of the first 8 patients, 5 had a PR, 2 SD (ORR = 63%).

- Phase II study combining cisplatin with TLK286.
  [Burris HA, *Proc Am Soc Clin Oncol* **23**: abstract 7126, 2005]
  - NSCLC patients with locally advanced or metastatic disease were treated with three escalating dose levels of TLK286 (750 or 1000 mg/m^2) and cisplatin (75 or 100 mg/m^2) q 3 weeks until disease progression or unacceptable toxicity.
  - TLK286 (1,000 mg/m^2) + cisplatin (75 mg/m^2), one level below the maximum tolerated dose (MTD) of 1,000/100 mg/m^2 of TLK286/cisplatin, showed grade 3 neutropenia in 2/5 patients, and this was chosen as the phase 2 dose.
  - Grade 3 neutropenia occurred in 28% of patients, and grade 3 thrombocytopenia in 4%.

- The ASSIST-2 (Assessment of Survival in Solid Tumors-2) clinical trial.
  - Compared TLK286 with gefitinib (Iressa), to find out if TLK286 ↑ survival in advanced NSCLC.
  - ASSIST-2 has enrolled 520 people, and the results are eagerly awaited.

- There is also a phase II trial in which TLK286 has been combined with docetaxel in platinum-resistant NSCLC; the results are pending.

Paclitaxel poliglumex (XYOTAX)

- Paclitaxel poliglumex (PPX) is a macromolecular drug conjugate that links paclitaxel with a biodegradable polymer, poly-L-glutamic acid.

- PPX is water soluble and can be administered as a 10-minute infusion, eliminating the need for cremophorEL ↓ the risk of hypersensitivity reactions, even without premedication.

- STELLAR 3 trial.
  [Langer CJ, *Proc Am Soc Clin Oncol* **23**: abstract 7011, 2005]
  - A phase III study randomizing stage IIIB/IV chemotherapy-naive NSCLC ECOG PS 2 patients to receive carboplatin (AUC = 6) and either PPX 210 mg/m^2 over 10 minutes or paclitaxel 225 mg/m^2 over 3 hours.
  - 400 patients were enrolled.
  - RESULTS:

- Survival was not significantly different between treatment groups (HR = 0.97).
- SIDE-EFFECTS:
  - Alopecia, arthralgias/myalgias, and cardiac events were significantly less frequent with PPX + carboplatin.
  - Hypersensitivity reactions did not occur more frequently with PPX, despite the lack of routine premedication.
  - Median time to neuropathy was 54 days for the paclitaxel + carboplatin group and 100 days for the PPX + carboplatin group ($p < 0.001$).

- STELLAR 4 trial.
  [Langer CJ, *Proc Am Soc Clin Oncol* 23(165 Pt I): abstract 7011, 2005]
  - Chemotherapy-naive population of PS 2 patients randomized.
    - PPX vs gentamicin or PPX vs vinorelbine.
  - RESULTS:
    - Median survival: 7.3 vs 6.6 months.
    - 1-year survival: 26% vs 28%.
    - PPX and gentamicin were equivalent; however, the vinorelbine group was statistically significantly inferior in median survival (6 months) and 1-year survival (7%) compared with the PPX group ($p = 0.012$, HR = 0.6).

- A pooled analysis of the results from the PPX-treated patients from the STELLAR 3 and 4 trials demonstrated a statistically significant ($p = 0.004$) survival advantage for ♀ treated when compared to ♂.
  - ♀ had a 39% probability of surviving at least 1 year vs 25% of ♂ (HR = 1.37; log rank, $p = 0.014$; $n = 463$ patients).

Oxaliplatin (Eloxatin)

[Cvitkovic E, *Br J Cancer* **77**(Suppl 4): 8–11, 1998]

- Oxaliplatin (*trans*-1-diaminocyclohexane-platinum) does not need preceding hydration; it does not carry a risk of nephropathy and there is minimal myelosuppression.

- The exact mechanism of action of oxaliplatin is currently unknown but, as with other platinum compounds, oxaliplatin causes the formation of DNA adducts that prevent DNA replication and transcription, which causes apoptosis.
  - In vitro studies have suggested that oxaliplatin is more potent than cisplatin, requiring fewer DNA adducts to attain an equal level of cytotoxicity.

Early studies with oxaliplatin in NSCLC

[Monnet I, *Eur J Cancer* **34**(7): 1124–1127, 1998]
[Monnet I, *J Clin Oncol* **19**(2): 458–463, 2001]
[Winegarden JD, *Ann Oncol* **15**: 915–920, 2004]

- From these 3 phase II studies we conclude the following.
  - Oxaliplatin has antitumor activity as a single agent in previously untreated advanced NSCLC, with an ORR of 15%.
  - The most common toxicity observed is transient and reversible, cold finger dysesthesia, which resolves within a few days in most cases.
  - The combination oxaliplatin + vinorelbine had an ORR = 37%, with a recommended dose of vinorelbine of 26 mg/m^2 and of oxaliplatin of 130 mg/m^2 on day 1 q 3 weeks.
  - The combination of oxaliplatin 130 mg/m^2 and paclitaxel 175 mg/m^2 every 21 days has an ORR of 34.2%, with 15.7% of patients experiencing grade 4 neutropenia, without any febrile episodes.

Combination of oxaliplatin with gemcitabine

[Franciosi V, *Lung Cancer* **41**(1): 101–106, 2003]
[Cappuzzo F, *J Clin Oncol* **23**(16s Pt I): abstract 3021, 2005]
[Bidoli P, *Proc Am Soc Clin Oncol* **23**: 648s (abstract 7118), 2005]
[Broad A, *Proc Am Soc Clin Oncol* **23**: 681s (abstract. 7244), 2005]

- These randomized, phase II studies show equivalency, validating the utility of oxaliplatin with gemcitabine in NSCLC.
  - One of the trials did not show activity; phase III trials are needed.

Combination of oxaliplatin with docetaxel or pemetrexed

- [Santos E, *Proc Am Soc Clin Oncol* **23**: 687s (abstract 7268), 2005]
  Reported safety and efficacy of the combination oxaliplatin + docetaxel, with a 37% ORR and 3% of grade 3/4 neutropenia, with the administration of 130 mg/m^2 and 70 mg/m^2, respectively, with routine use of pegfilgrastim.

- [Scagliotti GV, *Clin Cancer Res* **11**(2 Part 1): 690–696, 2005]
  First phase II, randomized, multicenter, clinical trial comparing pemetrexed + oxaliplatin vs carboplatin, showing equivalent results in the treatment of patients with advanced NSCLC.

- Phase III trials are needed.

Methylation inhibitors (azacytidine and decitabine)

The role of methylation in cancer

[Baylin SB, *Cancer Res* **46**(6): 2917–2922, 1986]
[Esteller M, *Cancer Res* **61**(8): 3225–3229, 2001]
[Zochbauer-Muller S, *Cancer Res* **61**(9): 3581–3585, 2001]

- Methylation of 'CpG islands', the promoter regions of many genes, has been linked to a loss of expression in vital genes.
  - Methylation is a frequently acquired epigenetic event in the pathogenesis of human cancers, including lung cancer.

Drugs targeting methylation

[Goffin J, *Ann Oncol* **13**(11): 1699–1716, 2002]
[Cheng JC, *J Natl Cancer Inst* **95**(5): 399–409, 2003]
[Thiagalingam S, *Ann N Y Acad Sci* **983**: 84–100, 2003]
[Marks PA, *Novartis Found Symp* **259**: 269–281, 2004]

- Drugs targeting methylation are: azacytidine, decitabine, fazarabine, and dihydro-5-azacytidine (DHAC).
  - Zebularine, antisense oligodeoxynucleotides, and histone deacetylase (HDAC) inhibitors are also being tried as agents targeting DNA methylation.
  - Only azacytidine and decitabine were found to have clinical efficacy.

Clinical trials including lung cancer patients

- [Schwartsmann G, *Invest New Drugs* **18**(1): 83–91, 2000]
  Phase I/II clinical trial using cisplatin + decitabine in 21 patients with solid tumors, including 8 with NSCLC, found the maximum tolerated dose (MTD) to be 120 mg/m^2 of decitabine, and dose-limiting toxicities (DLT) were neutropenia, thrombocytopenia, and mucositis.
  - There was one minor response in NSCLC.
- Phase II trial in 14 patients with NSCLC, who received cisplatin 33 mg/m^2 followed by decitabine 67 mg/m^2, both on days 1–3 q 3 weeks
  - Showed grade 3/4 neutropenia in 37%/23%, and grade 3/4 thrombocytopenia in 27%/13% of patients, respectively.
  - Only three minor responses were observed.

- Phase I–II study using decitabine in 15 patients with metastatic NSCLC.
  [Momparler RL, *Anticancer Drugs* **8**(4): 358–368, 1997]
  - Patients received decitabine 200–600 mg/m^2 by continuous infusion.
  - RESULTS:
    - Median survival → 6.7 months.
  - SIDE-EFFECTS:
    - Major side-effect → hematopoietic toxicity.

- [Williamson SK, *Invest New Drugs* **13**(1): 67–71, 1995]
  Phase II trial with fazarabine in 23 patients with NSCLC; no responses.

Lung cancer prevention

[Belinsky SA, *Nat Rev Cancer* **4**(9): 707–717, 2004]
[Fleming J, *Nutr Cancer* **40**(1): 42–49, 2001]
[Fiala ES, *Carcinogenesis* **19**(4): 597–604, 1998]

- Phase III clinical trial sponsored by the National Cancer Institute, in which 1,960 people will be randomized to determine whether 200 µg of L-selenomethionine given for 4 years can ↓ the incidence of secondary tumors in NSCLC patients who have undergone surgical resection for stage I disease.

- Selenium may prevent lung cancer, inhibiting cytosine DNA methyltransferase and acting as a demethylating agent.

Epothilones

Mechanism of action

[Bollag DM, *Cancer Res* **55**: 2325–2333, 1995]
[Kowalski RJ, *J Biol Chem* **272**: 2534–2541, 1997]
[Lee FY, *Clin Cancer Res* **7**: 1429–1437, 2001]
[Calvert PM, *Proc Am Soc Clin Oncol* **20**: abstract 429, 2001]

- Paclitaxel was the first product shown to promote tubulin assembly and stabilize microtubules.

- The epothilones were isolated from the myxobacterium *Sorangium cellulosum*, and were shown to have a similar mechanism of action.

- The epothilones are potential antitumor agents because they are effective against some multidrug-resistant cell lines that are resistant to paclitaxel.

– Some of them, like BMS-247550 (Ixabepilone), are twice as potent as paclitaxel in inducing tubulin polymerization.

Clinical studies including lung cancer patients

[Rubin EH, *Proc Am Soc Clin Oncol* **20**: abstract 270, 2001]
[Spriggs D, *Proc Am Soc Clin Oncol* **20**: abstract 42, 2001]
[LoRusso PM, *Proc Am Soc Clin Oncol* **20**: abstract 2125, 2001]
[Awada A, *Proc Am Soc Clin Oncol* **20**: abstract 427, 2001]
[Hao D, *Clin. Cancer Res* **7**: abstract 785, 2001]
[Mani S, *Proc Am Soc Clin Oncol***20**: abstract 269, 2001]
[Fojo AT, *Clin Cancer Res* **7**: abstract 774, 2001]

- Epothilone B has had diarrhea as DLT reported in two studies.

- Other grade 3 toxicities observed include fatigue, and nausea and vomiting.

- There are results from several phase I clinical trials with BMS-247550 used in several different schedules.
  – In general, DLTs have been seen with neuropathy, neutropenia, arthralgia, and myalgias.
  – Other reported toxicities are fatigue, weakness, constipation, diarrhea, nausea and vomiting, skin rash, alopecia, low-grade neuropathy, and anorexia.

- In the study by Spriggs there was 1 PR seen in NSCLC.

- [Yee L, *Proc Am Soc Clin Oncol* **23**: abstract 7127, 2005]
  A phase II study of KOS-862 (Epothilone D) as second-line therapy in NSCLC was reported, with only 1 PR and 2 SD among the 35 patients seen.

- [Shimizu T, *Proc Am Soc Clin Oncol* **23**: abstract 2050, 2005]
  Preliminary report of a Japanese, phase I study with Ixabepilone showed 8 SDs, including 3 patients with NSCLC among 13 patients.

Other drugs in development for NSCLC

[Pratesi G, *Anti-Cancer Drugs* **15**(6): 545–552, 2004]

- Gimatecan is a new topoisomerase I inhibitor that is administered orally; its main side-effect is hematopoietic toxicity.
  – Being studied in phase II trials for breast and lung cancer.

[Strumberg D, *J Clin Oncol* **23**: 965–972, 2005]
[Ratain MJ, *Proc Annu Meet Am Soc Clin Oncol* **23**: 4544, 2005]
[Escudier B, *Proc Annu Meet Am Soc Clin Oncol* **23**: LBA4510, 2005]

- Sorafenib (BAY 43–9006) is a novel oral Raf kinase and vascular endothelial growth factor receptor inhibitor.
  - Reported to have DLTs of diarrhea, fatigue, and skin toxicity, with 25 SD and one PR among 45 patients.
  - To date the drug has undergone phase III studies with very good results in renal cell carcinoma; phase II studies in NSCLC are ongoing.

- Similar agents, antiangiogenesis agents and tyrosine kinase inhibitors (TKIs) are reviewed more extensively in Chapter 18.

12

Surgery in small-cell lung cancer

- The role of surgery in small-cell lung cancer (SCLC) is controversial, even in limited disease.

- Surgery can be used in three instances:
  - Primary surgery followed by postoperative chemotherapy and, when indicated, mediastinal irradiation for tumors presenting as peripheral nodules.
  - Multimodality therapy, including induction chemotherapy followed by adjuvant surgery.
  - Salvage surgery.

- 16% of patients with SCLC are surgical candidates.

- Advantages of surgery: it may ↓ the frequency of local relapses; it does not influence the intensity of chemotherapy; it does not affect the bone marrow; and surgical staging may be of prognostic significance.

Surgery in limited-disease small-cell lung cancer

[Sridhar KS, *J Surg Oncol* **40**: 155–161, 1989]

- Primary surgical resection is definitely indicated in patients with $T_1N_0M_0$ lesions and probably in those with $T_1N_1M_0$ or $T_2N_0M_0$ lesions.

- If the tumor remains M_0 and resectable, a curative surgical approach similar to that in non-small-cell lung cancer (NSCLC) must be followed.

SCLC presenting as a solitary pulmonary nodule

- It is not unusual to find SCLC after excision/biopsy of a pulmonary nodule.

- It is common to undertake a diagnostic procedure (e.g. video-assisted thoracoscopy (VATS)) and a therapeutic procedure (lobectomy) at once when a solitary lesion is found.

- Surgical resection is the primary treatment of choice of a SCLC presenting as a solitary pulmonary nodule (SPN).
  [Kreisman H, *Chest* **101**: 225–231, 1992]

- SCLC presented as a SPN in 15 of 408 patients from 1979–1984.
  [Quoix E, *Cancer* **66**: 577–582, 1990]
  - 10 of the 15 patients with an SPN were resected, and 5 had chemotherapy and/or radiotherapy as primary treatment.
  - Postoperative chemotherapy was administered to most of the resected patients.
  - RESULTS:
    - Median survival of the 15 patients with an SPN → 24 months, which is significantly longer than other patients with SCLC.
    - A smaller initial tumor burden can improve the prognosis of patients with SCLC presenting as an SPN.

Role of surgery for bulky N_2 SCLC

[Kobayashi S, *Surg Today* **30**(11): 978–986, 2000]

- 30 consecutive patients with clinical stage III and pathologic stage III SCLC were reviewed, including 27 with N_2 disease who underwent surgery during the period 1982–1992. Of these, 7 (23%) survived disease-free for over 5 years.

- Combined-modality therapy, based on a sensitivity assay in vitro, was given.

- The cell characteristics in vitro and the actual treatment of 5 patients with bulky N_2 lesions were examined (4 of whom were long-term survivors and 1 of whom died 11 months after surgery) as controls for comparison with the long-term survivors.

- Based on the results of the cell characteristics in vitro, SCLC was determined to be a heterogeneous tumor.

- Surgical excision of the primary tumor with adjuvant therapy might be necessary to achieve long-term survival and maintain good performance status, and to improve quality of life in patients with bulky N_2 SCLC, eliminating drug-resistant tumor cells within the primary tumor.

Surgery after induction chemotherapy

- Available data come from phase II trials with relatively small numbers of patients in each trial.

- [Shepherd FA, *Comprehensive Textbook in Thoracic Oncology*, Williams & Wilkins, Baltimore, OH, pp. 439–455, 1996]
  - Review of 9 phase II trials of surgical resection following induction chemotherapy.
  - 260 patients with SCLC.
  - The chemotherapy response → at least 88% in 8 of the 9 trials.
  - 60% of patients underwent surgery, and in 80% of these complete resection was achieved.
  - Most of the resected patients had viable residual SCLC in the resection specimen with a pathologic complete response in → 10%.
  - In patients with pathological stage I disease who underwent complete resection, the 5-year survival was ~ 70%.
    - However, in patients with stage II or III, survival was not impressive.

- Randomized trial.
  [Lad T, *Chest* **106**: 320S–323S, 1994]
  - Prospective randomized trial to determine benefit of surgical resection of residual disease following induction chemotherapy.
  - After induction chemotherapy, 146 patients were randomized to either surgical resection followed by thoracic and prophylactic cranial irradiation (PCI), or thoracic radiation and PCI.
  - RESULTS:
    - No significant difference was found between the two groups in either median or long-term survival.
    - It was not possible to determine survival based on tumor stage or TNM classification because complete pathological staging was done only in patients who underwent surgery.
    - Furthermore, 10% of the patients did not receive the protocol-specified therapy ,and many patients with T_3 or N_2 tumors were included.

- [Shepherd FA, *J Thorac Cardiovasc Surg* **97**: 177–186, 1989]
  - Retrospective study.

- 119 SCLC patients treated with pre- or postoperative chemotherapy and surgery.
- RESULTS:
  - Proper staging identifies patients with an excellent prognosis.
  - Patients with stage I disease had a 5-year survival of 51%.
  - Survival of those with stage II and IIIA disease was similar to that of patients with NSCLC treated surgically.

Salvage surgery

[Shepherd FA, *J Thorac Cardiovasc Surg* **101**: 196–200, 1991]
[Elliot JA, *J Clin Oncol* **5**: 246–254, 1987]

- Surgery for SCLC persisting in the primary site after primary non-surgical treatment or recurring only in the primary site following a complete response.

- A small number of patients with limited SCLC without mediastinal node involvement may be cured by surgery after relapse or failure to respond to chemotherapy and radiotherapy.

- Residual disease at the primary tumor site was found in only 31% of the patients after radical resection, but in 92% of patients without resection but a negative mediastinoscopy.

- The average number of tumor-involved sites at autopsy was 2.5 in the resection group and 4.2 in the non-resected group.

- The chest remains the most frequent site of recurrent disease, even in patients with initially limited disease.

13

Chemotherapy in limited-disease, small-cell lung cancer

[Turrisi A, *N Engl J Med* **340**: 265–271, 1999]

- Limited-disease, small-cell lung cancer (LD-SCLC) is defined as disease limited to one hemithorax and encompassable within a single radiation port.

- A median survival of 23 months and a 5-year survival of 26% have been reported for combined modality chemotherapy with etoposide + cisplatin (EP) and twice daily radiotherapy to 45 Gy.

- Four to six cycles of chemotherapy in the management of LD-SCLC and extensive-disease, small-cell lung cancer (ED-SCLC) appear to be optimal.
  [DeVita V, *Cancer Principles & Practice of Oncology*, 7th edn, Philadelphia, Lippincott Williams and Wilkins, 2005, p. 819]
  - Maintenance chemotherapy beyond induction is of unproven value.

- Cyclophosphamide + doxorubicin + vincristine (CAV) was the standard in the management of SCLC.
  [Livingstone RB, *Ann Intern Med* **88**: 194–199, 1978]
  - CAV was given in a sequential fashion with radiation to the primary tumor and brain to 358 patients with SCLC (ED-SCLC in 250, LD-SCLC in 108).
  - A median survival of 13 months and an overall response rate (ORR) of 75%, with 41% of complete responses, for patients with LD-SCLC were observed.

- Systematic review of 36 trials.
  [Mascaux C, *Lung Cancer* **30**: 23–36, 2000]
  - 1980–1998: nine of the trials (total of 1,945 patients) compared systemic regimens including EP with regimens using neither cisplatin nor etoposide.
  - EP resulted in a highly significant benefit compared to regimens not containing either drug: hazard ratio 0.57 (95% CI, 0.51–0.64) ($p < 0.001$).

- Randomized, phase III trial, wherein 436 patients with ED-SCLC and LD-SCLC were randomized to either EP or cyclophosphamide + epirubicin + vincristine (CEV).
  [Sundstrom S, *J Clin Oncol* **20**: 4665–4672, 2002]
  - RESULTS:
    - Among LD-SCLC patients, the median survival time was 14.5 months with EP and 9.7 months with CEV ($p = 0.001$).
    - In addition, the 2- and 5-year survival rates favored EP (25%) over CEV (10%) ($p = 0.0001$).
    - No difference in survival was observed among patients with ED-SCLC.

- Small, randomized trial including 61 ED-SCLC patients and 82 LD-SCLC patients.
  [Kosmidis PA, *Semin Oncol* **21**(3 Suppl 6): 23–30, 1994]
  - Carboplatin 300 mg/m^2 on day 1; cisplatin 50 mg/m^2 on days 1 and 2.
  - Both groups received etoposide 100 mg/m^2 daily ×3 days.
  - Cycles repeated every 3 weeks.
  - In LD-SCLC patients, radiation was given concomitantly with chemotherapy.
  - RESULTS:
    - ORR, median survival, and 2-year survival were not different overall or in LD-SCLC patients in the two groups.
  - CONCLUSIONS:
    - Carboplatin may be considered as a substitute for cisplatin in patients with poor performance status.
    - However, in our opinion cisplatin should be preferred over carboplatin whenever possible in LD-SCLC patients where cure is the primary objective of therapy.

- Randomized, phase III trial including LD-SCLC and ED-SCLC patients, testing the addition of paclitaxel to EP (TEP) vs EP alone.
  [Mavroudis D, *Ann Oncol* **12**: 463–470, 2001]

- The trial was terminated early due to excess toxicity in the TEP group.
- 62 patients received 261 cycles of TEP and 71 patients received 323 cycles of EP.
- RESULTS:
  - The duration of response, 1-year survival and overall survival were similar in the two groups.
  - In an intention-to-treat subgroup analysis of patients with LD-SCLC there was no difference in efficacy between the two regimens.
- SIDE-EFFECTS:
  - There were eight toxic deaths in the TEP group vs none in the EP group ($p = 0.001$).
  - More grade 4 neutropenia and febrile neutropenia (despite use of granulocyte colony stimulating factor), grade 3–4 thrombocytopenia, grade 3–4 diarrhea, grade 3–4 asthenia, and grade 3 neurotoxicity were observed in the TEP group.

- The results of this trial are similar to the intergroup effort studying the addition of paclitaxel to EP (TEP) vs EP alone in ED-SCLC.
  [Niell HB, *J Clin Oncol* **23**: 3752–3759, 2005]

In summary:

- The standard of care for ED-SCLC remains platinum based chemotherapy with etoposide and concomitant radiation.
  - Other chemotherapeutic agents, such as irinotecan, are being tested in this setting.

14

Radiation therapy for limited-disease, small-cell lung cancer

[Turrisi A, *Curr Treat Options Oncol* **4**(1): 61–64, 2003]
[Kaminsky JM, *Chest Surg Clin N Am* **13**(1): 149–167, 2003]
[Raez LE, *Curr Treat Options Oncol* **6**(1): 69–74, 2005]

- There is a lower rate of chest relapse with combined modality therapy.
  - Nevertheless, local recurrence still approaches → 33%.

- The use of combined modality ↑ the toxicity of therapy, but the 2-year disease survival appears superior for combined modality therapy.

Fallacies in study design

- There are many fallacies in the design of studies of combined modality therapy for limited-disease lung cancer:
  - Heterogeneous definition of local relapse.
  - Variations in radiation dose and schedule.
  - Variation in radiation fields.
  - Variation in dose per fraction.
  - Use of specific chemotherapy programs.
  - Use of less than optimal chemotherapy.
  - Use of less than optimal radiation therapy (XRT).

Why is thoracic radiation needed?

- Small-cell lung cancer (SCLC) is the most sensitive cell type of lung cancer to radiation.

- Objective tumor regression occurs in > 90% of treated patients.

- The primary tumor bed is the site of progression in up to 80% of relapsing patients treated with chemotherapy alone.

Sequencing of radiation therapy with chemotherapy

- The sequencing of chemotherapy and XRT is Not Standardized.

- Three ways of sequencing chemotherapy and XRT have been described.
  - **Concurrent**: chemotherapy and XRT are given at the same time.
  - **Alternating**: XRT is given on days when no chemotherapy is delivered, in a cyclic fashion.
  - **Sequential**: one modality is delivered after the other has been completed.

Early randomized trials: concurrent treatment

- [Perry MC, *N Engl J Med* **316**: 912–918, 1987]
  - 399 evaluable patients.
  - Concurrent treatment vs delayed XRT (after 3 cycles) vs chemotherapy only.
  - Multi-agent chemotherapy was used:
    - vincristine, cyclophosphamide (Cytoxan), doxorubicin (Adriamycin) and etoposide.
  - XRT:
    - Standard fractionation was given to a total dose of 5000 cGy.
    - Radiation fields were large and all patients received prophylactic cranial irradiation (PCI).
- [Bunn P, *Ann Intern Med* **106**: 655–602, 1987]
  - 96 evaluable patients.
  - Concurrent treatment vs chemotherapy alone.
  - Multiagent chemotherapy was used:
    - cyclophosphamide (Cytoxan), methotrexate, and CCNU.
  - XRT:
    - 266.67 cGy/fraction was given to a total dose of 4000 cGy.
    - Radiation fields encompassed visible disease only, and all patients received PCI.

Early randomized trials: alternating treatment

- [Perez CA, *J Clin Oncol* **2**: 1200–1208, 1984]
  - 291 evaluable patients.

- Alternating treatment vs chemotherapy alone.
- Multiagent chemotherapy was used:
  - cyclophosphamide (Cytoxan), doxorubicin (Adriamycin), and vincristine.
- XRT:
  - 285.71 cGy/fraction was given to a total dose of 4000 cGy.
  - Radiation fields were large.

Early randomized trials: sequential treatment

- [Fox T, *Int J Radiat Oncol Biol Phys* **6**: 1083, 1980]
  - Sequential treatment vs chemotherapy alone.
  - Multiagent chemotherapy was used:
    - cyclophosphamide (Cytoxan), doxorubicin (Adriamycin), methotrexate, and etoposide.
- XRT:
  - Standard fractionation was given to a total dose of 4000 cGy.
  - Radiation fields were large.

Summary of early randomized trials

| Author | *p* | Median survival (months) | | 2-year DFS or OS (%) | |
		CT	CMT	CT	CMT
Bunn	0.035	11.6	15	12	28 (OS)
Perry	0.009	13.6	13.1/14.6	8	15/25 (DFS)
Perez	0.03	11.2	14	19	28 (OS)
Fox	0.003	12.7	16.5	2	15 (DFS)

CMT, combined modality therapy; CT, chemotherapy alone; DFS, disease-free survival; OS, overall survival.

Summary of negative randomized trials

[Osterlind K, *Br J Cancer* **54**: 7–17, 1986]
[Souhami RL, *BMJ* **288**: 1643–1646, 1984]
[Kies MS, *J Clin Oncol* **5**: 592–600, 1987]

- Three randomized trials <u>did not</u> show improvement in survival.
  - Of these three, one used concurrent therapy and two used sequential therapy.

Meta-analyses

[Pignon JP, *N Engl J Med* **327**: 1618–1624, 1992]
[Warde P, *J Clin Oncol* **10**: 890–895, 1992]

- Two meta-analyses have examined the available studies to determine whether the addition of thoracic XRT to systemic chemotherapy improves 2-year survival and local control.
  - > 2,100 patients with limited-stage SCLC, randomized to receive chemotherapy alone or chemotherapy + XRT, were included in these meta-analyses.
- RESULTS:
  - 14% ↓ in death rate due to disease.
  - 5.4% improvement in 3-year survival.
  - Both differences were highly statistically significant in favor of combined modality therapy.

Early vs late thoracic radiation

Randomized trials

- [Perry MC, *N Engl J Med* **316**: 912–918, 1987]
  - This study not only evaluated if there was a benefit in survival by adding thoracic XRT to chemotherapy in limited-stage SCLC (see early randomized trials of concurrent treatment) but also evaluated the potential benefit of adding XRT early in the course of treatment.
  - RESULTS:
    - A 2-year DFS of 15% for early thoracic radiation vs 25% for late thoracic radiation.

- [Murray N, *J Clin Oncol* **11**: 336–344, 1993]
  - Compared early (week 3) vs late (week 15) thoracic XRT in 308 patients.
  - Multiagent chemotherapy was used:
    - cyclophosphamide (Cytoxan) + doxorubicin (Adriamycin) + vincristine (CAV) alternating with etoposide + cisplatin (EP).
  - Radiation dose:
    - 40 Gy in 15 fractions/3 weeks using moderately sized radiation fields.
  - All patients received PCI.
  - RESULTS:
    - OS → 21.2% for early XRT vs 16% for late XRT.

- – Median progression-free survival (PFS) → 15.4% for early XRT vs 11.8% for late XRT.
- – 3-year PFS → 26% for early XRT vs 19% for late XRT.
- – All values are statistically significant, but the overall response was not statistically significant.

- [Work E, *J Clin Oncol* **15**: 3030–3037, 1997]
  - 199 patients, early vs late (18-week delay) thoracic XRT.
  - Multiagent chemotherapy was used:
    - – cyclophosphamide (Cytoxan) + doxorubicin (Adriamycin) + vincristine (CAV) alternating with etoposide + cisplatin (EP).
  - XRT:
    - – Dose: 40 or 45 Gy, using standard fractionation.
    - – Delivered using a split course.
    - – Radiation fields included visible disease only and all patients received PCI.
  - RESULTS:
    - – 2-year OS → 20% (early XRT) vs 19% (late XRT); $p = 0.4$.
    - – 2-year in-field recurrence → 72% (early XRT) vs 68% (late XRT); $p = 0.2$.
    - – Median survival → 10.5 months (early XRT) vs 12.0 months (late XRT).
  - LIMITATIONS OF THE STUDY:
    - – Split course radiation is not considered standard in XRT for SCLC.
    - – Chemotherapy was not given concomitantly with XRT.
    - – First radiation dose (40 Gy) is considered too low (high intra-thoracic failure rate).
    - – Today, in many academic centers hyperfractionation is the preferred approach to thoracic radiation, as SCLC has a high growth fraction, a short cell-cycle time, and a small to absent shoulder in cell survival curves.
    - – Why is the 2-year survival so low (~ 20%) in both groups?

Hyperfractionation in SCLC

- [Turrisi A, *N Engl J Med* **340**: 265–271, 1999]
  - 417 patients with limited-stage disease randomized to 45 Gy at 1.8 Gy/fraction, 1 fraction/day vs 45 Gy at 1.5 Gy/fraction, 2 fraction/day.
  - Median follow-up → 5 years.

- RESULTS:

	Once daily	Twice daily	p
Local failure (%)	52	36	0.06
Loca failure + distant metastases (%)	23	6	0.01
Overall survival (%)	16	26	0.04

- SIDE-EFFECTS:
  - Overall morbidities were no different between the two groups.
  - Higher frequency of grade III esophagitis with the twice daily treatment.
- LIMITATIONS OF THE STUDY:
  - The study was criticized because 45 Gy twice daily is not widely accepted; a lot of centers use higher doses (> 50 Gy) in the more standard once daily fashion, with good results.
  - Ongoing randomized studies will resolve this issue.

Prophylactic cranial irradiation

[Hansen H, *Cancer* **46**: 279–284, 1980]
[Aroney RS, *Cancer Treat Rep* **67**: 675–682, 1983]
[Beiler D, *Int J Radiat Oncol Biol Phys* **5**: 941, 1979]
[Cox JD, *Cancer* **42**: 1135–1140, 1978]
[Eagan RT, *Cancer Clin Trial* **4**: 261–266, 1981]
[Jackson DV, *JAMA* **237**: 2730–2733, 1977]
[Seydel HG, *Am J Clin Oncol* **8**: 218, 1985]
[Niiranen A, *Acta Oncol* **28**: 501, 1989]
[Kristjansen PE, *Lung Cancer* **12**: S23, 1995]

- 11 randomized trials that evaluated the potential benefit of PCI.

- It is known that brain metastasis are detected in ∼ 10% of patients with SCLC at presentation.

- 20–25% are subsequently diagnosed with brain metastasis.

- The probability of brain metastasis if no brain XRT is given is approximately 50–80%.

- Postmortem series show up to 65% incidence of brain metastasis.
  - RESULTS:
    - A significant clinical ↓ in detectable brain metastasis is achieved from 24% → 6% but with no effect on survival.

[Auperin A, *N Engl J Med* **341**: 476, 1999]
- Retrospectively evaluated the use of PCI in complete responders with (limited-stage disease).
  - RESULTS:
    - Suggested a survival benefit of PCI only in complete responders.

- Actuarial analysis.
  [Rosen ST, *Am J Med* **74**: 615, 1983]
  [Aroney RS, *Cancer Treat Rep* **67**: 675, 1983]
  - Partial response or no response are associated with similar risks of recurrence in the brain, regardless of whether PCI was administered.

- Meta-analyses for PCI.
  [Arriagada R, *J Natl Cancer Inst* **87**: 766, 1995]
  [Gregor A, *Eur J Cancer* **33**: 1752, 1997]
  [Meyers CA, *Lung Cancer* **12**: 231, 1995]
  - Included 1,000 patients in 7 trials that evaluated patients with complete response to combined modality therapy randomized to receive PCI or not.
  - RESULTS:
    - A significant ↑ in survival for complete responders was seen in those who received PCI (21% vs 15% at 3 years).
    - PCI did significantly ↓ the probability of brain metastasis or ↑ the likelihood of DFS.
  - LIMITATIONS OF THE STUDY:
    - There was no assessment of cognitive function, as most studies did not include a baseline assessment.

Toxicity of PCI

[Crossen JR, *J Clin Oncol* **12**(3): 627–642, 1994]

- Cognitive and neuropsychometric testing abnormalities have been described in patients who received PCI.
  - These abnormalities are more prominent in patients who received high dose per fraction PCI with concurrent chemotherapy.

- Not all deficits are due to radiation.

- Other contributing factors include:
  - Alcohol.
  - Smoking.
  - Chemotherapy.
  - Paraneoplastic syndromes.

- Encephalopathy.
  Historical overview of 18 studies of PCI that include neurobehavioral reports and XRT parameters.
  - 16/18 studies involving SCLC patients.
  - 96/364 patients evaluated in the 16 studies had encephalopathy due to PCI.
  - LIMITATIONS OF THE STUDY:
    - Computerized tomography (CT) rather than magnetic resonance imaging (MRI) was used in patient evaluation.
    - Neurobehavioral abnormalities were generally underestimated.

- Mechanisms of brain injury.
  - Immunologic process akin to allergic reaction from antigen released from damaged glial cells, resulting in vascular damage, and occlusion and demyelination.
    - White matter is the most vulnerable target of the injury.
  - Vascular injury to small- and medium-sized blood vessels of the brain.
    - This is the basis of radionecrosis, but is not clearly the basis of neurobehavioral abnormality.

- Doses used for PCI usually varied from 24 to 40 Gy; the modal fraction size was 3 Gy in 10 fractions.

- Variables affecting subclinical and clinical brain injuries include PCI dose, fraction size, chemotherapeutic effect, and sequencing and timing of chemotherapy and XRT.

- [Johnson BE, *J Clin Oncol* **8**(1): 48–56, 1990]
  - 20/360 new SCLC patients were alive with no evidence of disease 4 years after PCI was given. Neurological follow-up was done in these survivors.
  - 16 were still alive at the time of the study, and 15 returned for follow-up.
  - RESULTS:
    - 9/16 patients returned to a lifestyle comparable to that before their treatment for SCLC.
    - 13/15 patients had neurologic complaints.
    - 10/15 had an abnormal neurologic examination.
    - 7/14 had an abnormal mental status examination.
    - 12/14 had abnormal neuropsychologic testing.
    - 12/15 had abnormal CT scans.
    - 7/15 had white matter abnormalities on MRI scans.

- There was no further ↓ in performance status, functional status, neurologic symptoms, or neurologic examination in these 16 survivors of 13 years with the additional 4 years of follow-up.

Recommendations for PCI

- Avoid concurrent chemotherapy and XRT.

- Delay PCI until at least 1 week after chemotherapy has been completed.

- Most common time of onset of central nervous system toxicities is 6–24 months after PCI.

- Systematic long-term studies with pre- and post-PCI neurologic examination, neuropsychiatric testing, and performance status assessment is recommended.

15

Extensive-disease, small-cell lung cancer

- ~ 2/3 of patients with small-cell lung cancer (SCLC) are diagnosed with extensive-disease, small-cell lung cancer (ED-SCLC).

- Rarely curable; the main goal is palliation.

- The treatment is primarily chemotherapy.

- Thoracic radiotherapy (XRT) is not routinely used in ED-SCLC, except for palliation of locoregional complications, such as severe pain, airway obstruction, or hemoptysis.

Chemotherapy agents

[Chute JP, *J Clin Oncol* **17**: 1794–1801, 1999]
[Mascaux C, *Lung Cancer* **30**: 23–36, 2000]
[Pujol JL, *Br J Cancer* **83**: 8–15, 2000]

- Cyclophosphamide, doxorubicin (Adriamycin), vincristine, etoposide, topotecan, irinotecan, paclitaxel, docetaxel, and gemcitabine.

- Monotherapy has response rates (RRs) > 30%.

- RRs for combination chemotherapy are usually 50% or higher.

- The median survival time ranges from 8 to 12 months.

- Combination chemotherapy is superior to monotherapy with respect to survival.

First-line chemotherapy for extensive-disease, small-cell lung cancer

- Cisplatin or carboplatin + etoposide is the most common regimen used.
- Carboplatin appears to have similar efficacy and is better tolerated than cisplatin.

Table 15.1 Most common regimens used for first-line treatment of ED-SCLC

Dosage	Frequency
Cisplatin 80 mg/m^2 on day 1 + etoposide 100 mg/m^2 on days 1–3 [Schiller JH, *J Clin Oncol* **19**: 2114–2122, 2001]	q 3 weeks
Cisplatin 60 mg/m^2 on day 1 + irinotecan 60 mg/m^2 on days 1, 8, and 15 [Sandler A, *Proc Am Soc Clin Oncol* **22**: 631 (abstract 2537), 2003]	q 4 weeks
Carboplatin (AUC = 5) on day 1 + etoposide 100 mg/m^2 on days 1–5 (p.o.) [Larive S, *Lung Cancer* **35**(1): 1–7, 2002]	q 4 weeks

- Ongoing trials are evaluating the combination of cisplatin + irinotecan as an alternative to cisplatin + etoposide.
- Randomized, phase III, intergroup trial of etoposide + cisplatin with or without paclitaxel and granulocyte colony-stimulating factor (GCSF).
  [Niell HB, *J Clin Oncol* **23**(16): 3752–3759, 2005]
  - 587 untreated patients randomized.
    - Group I: cisplatin 80 mg/m^2 on day 1 + etoposide 80 mg/m^2 on days 1–3 q 3 weeks for 6 cycles (EP).
    - Group II: cisplatin 80 mg/m^2 on day 1 + paclitaxel 175 mg/m^2 on day 1 + etoposide 80 mg/m^2 on days 1–3 followed by GCSF on days 4–18 q 3 weeks for 6 cycles (PET).
  - RESULTS:
    - RR → 68% for EP group, 75% for PET group.

- Median failure-free survival time → 5.9 months for EP, 6 months for PET ($p = 0.179$).
  - Median overall survival (OS) → 9.9 months for EP, 10.6 months for PET ($p = 0.169$).
- SIDE-EFFECTS:
  - Toxic deaths occurred in 2.4% in EP group and 6.5% in PET group.
- CONCLUSIONS:
  - PET did not improve time to progression (TTP) or OS in patients with extensive SCLC compared with EP alone, and was associated with unacceptable toxicity.
  - The use of triplet therapy cannot be recommended at this time.

- **Comparison of combined irinotecan + cisplatin (IP) and conventional cisplatin + etoposide (EP).**
  [Noda K, *N Engl J Med* **346**: 85–91, 2002]
  - Multicenter, randomized, phase III study of 154 patients with ED-SCLC.
  - The planned study size was 230 patients, but enrolment was terminated early because of a statistically significant difference in survival between the IP and EP groups.
  - RESULTS:
    - Median survival → 12.8 months for IP, 9.4 months for EP ($p = 0.002$).
    - 2-year survival → 19.5% for IP, 5.2% for EP.
  - SIDE-EFFECTS:
    - Severe myelosuppression was more frequent with EP, and severe diarrhea was more frequent with IP.
  - CONCLUSIONS:
    - IP is an effective treatment for ED-SCLC.
    - Two confirmatory trials have been started in the USA to validate these results.

- **Irinotecan + cisplatin (IP) vs etoposide + cisplatin (EP) in patients with previously untreated ED-SCLC.**
  [Hanna NH, *Proc Am Soc Clin Oncol* **23**(622s): abstract 7004, 2005]
  - Multicenter, open-label, randomized, phase III trial.
  - 300 patients accrued (221 IP; 110 EP).
  - The primary endpoint was OS.
  - Cisplatin 30 mg/m^2 + irinotecan 65 mg/m^2 on days 1 and 8 q 21 days or cisplatin 60 mg/m^2 on day 1 + etoposide 120 mg/m^2 i.v. on days 1–3 q 21 days ×4 cycles.

- RESULTS:
  - No statistically significant difference between IP and EP in RR (52% vs 51%), median TTP (4.1 vs 4.6 months), median survival (9.3 vs 10.2 months), or 1-year survival (35% vs 36.1%).
- SIDE-EFFECTS:
  - Grade 3/4 toxicities for IP and EP were: neutropenia (36% vs 86%), febrile neutropenia (4% vs 10%), anemia (5% vs 11%), thrombocytopenia (4% vs 19%), and diarrhea (21% vs 0%).
- CONCLUSIONS:
  - No significant difference in OS.
  - Patients receiving IP had less myelosuppression but more diarrhea than patients receiving EP.

- **Irinotecan + carboplatin (PI) vs etoposide + carboplatin (PE) in ED-SCLC.**
  [Schmittel A, *Proc Am Soc Clin Oncol* **23**: abstract 7046, 2005]
  - Randomized, phase II trial of 74 chemotherapy-naive patients.
  - Carboplatin (AUC = 5) + irinotecan 50 mg/m^2 on days 1, 8, and 15 q 4 weeks, or + etoposide 140 mg/m^2 on days 1–3 q 3 weeks.
  - RESULTS:
    - Complete response/partial response/stable disease/progression of disease was observed in 10%/61%/6%/23% with PI and 0%/50%/11%/43% with PE.
  - SIDE-EFFECT:
    - Grade 3 and 4 toxicity was observed for thrombocytopenia (18% PI vs 50% PE) and neutropenia (27% PI vs 62% PE).
  - CONCLUSION:
    - PI improves RR and progression-free survival (PFS) over standard PE.

- **Oral topotecan + cisplatin (TC) vs i.v. etoposide + cisplatin (PE) as treatment for chemotherapy-naive patients with ED-SCLC.**
  [Eckardt J, *Proc Am Soc Clin Oncol* **23**(621s): abstract 7003, 2005]
  - 859 patients were recruited.
  - Randomized, phase III trial to compare safety and efficacy in this setting.
  - Oral topotecan 1.7 mg/m^2 on days 1–5 + cisplatin 60 mg/m^2 on day 5, or + etoposide 100 mg/m^2 i.v. on days 1–3 and cisplatin 80 mg/m^2 on day 1.
  - Baseline characteristics were balanced.
  - RESULTS:
    - Median number of cycles (range) for TC was 5 (1–9), and for PE was 6 (1–8).

    – TC and PE were well tolerated.
- SIDE-EFFECTS:
  - Neutropenia was more common with EP.
  - Thrombocytopenia and anemia were more common with TC.
- CONCLUSION:
  - TC and PE show comparable activity and tolerability.

- **Maintenance or 'consolidation' chemotherapy.**
  [Schiller JH, *J Clin Oncol* **19**: 2114–2122, 2001]
  - ECOG 7593, phase III clinical trial.
  - 425 patients with ED-SCLC received 4 cycles of EP q 3 weeks.
  - 227 patients achieved a response or disease stabilization and were randomized to observation or up to 6 cycles of topotecan 1.5 mg/m^2 daily for 5 days q 3 weeks.
  - RESULTS:
    - Objective RR → 7% to consolidation topotecan, and no impact on survival was observed (8.9 vs 9.3 months; $p = 0.43$).
    - PFS was significantly better with topotecan compared with observation (3.6 vs 2.3 months; $p < 0.001$).
  - SIDE-EFFECT:
    - 22% grade 3/4 anemia in topotecan group, with no difference in quality of life.
  - CONCLUSIONS:
    - 4 cycles of EP induction therapy followed by 4 cycles of topotecan improved PFS, but not OS or quality of life in ED-SCLC.
    - Maintenance is not currently recommended.

Second-line therapy for extensive-disease, small-cell lung cancer

[Ardizzoni A, *J Clin Oncol* **15**: 2090–2096, 1997]

- Despite a good RR with initial chemotherapy, most patients will relapse.

- Patients are often symptomatic at relapse and require immediate palliation.

- Patients who relapse > 90 days after first-line therapy are said to have sensitive disease.

- Patients who relapse within 90 days are described as having resistant disease, and have a worse prognosis than patients with sensitive disease.

- Several agents have been studied for the second-line treatment of SCLC.

- Topotecan is the only approved treatment in this setting.

Table 15.2   Most common regimens used for second-line treatment of ED-SCLC

Dosage	Frequency
Topotecan 1.25–1.5 mg/m² on days 1–5	q 3 weeks
[von Pawel J, *J Clin Oncol* **17**: 658–667, 1999]	
Topotecan 4 mg/m² weekly	For 12 weeks
[Greco FA, *Lung Cancer* **41**(Suppl 4): 9–16, 2003]	

- **Combination chemotherapy vs topotecan monotherapy for relapsed ED-SCLC.**
  [Von Pawel J, *J Clin Oncol* **17**: 658–667, 1999]
  - Randomized, multicenter study of 211 patients with SCLC that relapsed at least 60 days after completion of first-line therapy.
  - Patients received either topotecan 1.5 mg/m² daily for 5 days q 21 days, or cyclophosphamide 1,000 mg/m² + doxorubicin 45 mg/m² + vincristine 2 mg (CAV) infused on day 1 q 21 days.
  - RESULTS:
    - RR: 24.3% with topotecan, 18.3% with CAV ($p = 0.285$).
    - TTP: 13.3 weeks for topotecan, 12.3 weeks for CAV ($p = 0.552$).
    - Median survival: 25 weeks for topotecan, 24.7 weeks for CAV ($p = 0.795$).
    - Symptom improvement was greater in the topotecan group ($p \leq 0.043$).
  - SIDE-EFFECTS:
    - Grade 4 thrombocytopenia and grade 3/4 anemia occurred more frequently with topotecan (9.8% and 17.7% vs 1.4% and 7.2%, respectively) ($p < 0.001$).
  - CONCLUSIONS:
    - Topotecan was at least as effective as CAV in the treatment of patients with recurrent SCLC and resulted in greater symptom improvement.

- Diminishing myelosuppression associated with topotecan.
  - The US Food and Drug Administration approved dose of topotecan (1.5 mg/m^2 daily ×5 days) is always difficult to tolerate. Several options include reducing the dose or reducing the number of days of therapy.
  - Weekly administration represents a good alternative.
  - **Weekly topotecan in the second-line treatment of SCLC.**
    [Greco FA, *Lung Cancer* **41**(Suppl 2): S237, 2003]
    - Phase II trial of topotecan 4 mg/m2 q week ×12.
    - 12 patients enrolled.
    - SIDE-EFFECTS:
      - 2 patients with grade 3–4 thrombocytopenia, and 1 patient with grade 3 leukopenia and neutropenia.
      - No grade 3–4 non-hematologic toxicity reported.
    - CONCLUSION:
      - Weekly topotecan may be better tolerated than the classic 5-day schedule.

- **Comparing single-agent etoposide with combination chemotherapy in patients with poor performance status.**
  [Girling DJ, Medical Research Council Trial, *Lancet* **348**: 563–566, 1996]
  - Etoposide p.o. vs one of two i.v. combination regimens (EV and CAV) in patients with poor performance status.
  - 339 patients were randomized.
  - RESULTS:
    - Interim analysis showed an improved median survival in favor of the i.v. group (183 vs 130 days, $p = 0.03$).
    - Palliative effects after 3 months of therapy were slightly superior in the i.v. group (46% vs 41%).

- Etoposide p.o. vs combination chemotherapy in patients with poor performance status or > 75 years of age with limited-disease SCLC (LD-SCLC) or ED-SCLC.
  [Clark PI, *Proc Am Soc Clin Oncol* **16**: abstract 1124, 1996]
  - RESULTS:
    - Improved survival and quality of life with the standard chemotherapy regimen, consistent with the results of the above Medical Research Council trial.
  - CONCLUSION:
    - Based on these studies, patients with poor prognostic features appear to derive greater benefit from combination regimens compared to single-agent therapy.

Other chemotherapeutic options for extensive-disease, small-cell lung cancer

[Rushing DA, *Proc Am Soc Clin Oncol* 18: 484a, 1999]
[Agelaki S, *Eur J Cancer* 35: S258, 1999]
[Lassen U, *Proc Am Soc Clin Oncol* 23: 664a, 2004]
[Dongiovanni V, *Proc Am Soc Clin Oncol* 23: 665a, 2004]
[Lusch G, *Proc Am Soc Clin Oncol* 18: 478a, 1999]
[Masuda N, *J Clin Oncol* 16: 3329–3334, 1998]

- ED-SCLC or relapsed or refractory SCLC have a uniformly poor prognosis.

- Several small, phase II studies of various combination chemotherapy regimens have been reported as options for the treatment of ED-SCLC.
  - Including irinotecan + etoposide, oral etoposide + hexamethylmelamine, irinotecan + paclitaxel, carboplatin + paclitaxel, and paclitaxel + gemcitabine.
  - RESULTS:
    - RRs ranged from 17% to 71%, but median survival still ranged from 7.4 to 36 weeks with no significant difference according to the actual standard therapy mentioned above.

[Zangemeister-Wittke U, *Br J Cancer* 78(8): 1035–1042, 1998]
[Rudin CM, *Ann Oncol* 13(4): 539–545, 2002]
[Shepard FA, *J Clin Oncol* 20(22): 4434–4439, 2002]
[Socinski MA, *Proc Am Soc Clin Oncol* 23: 664a, 2004]

- Marimastat (a matrix metalloproteinase inhibitor) used in consolidation chemotherapy for SCLC failed to show a survival benefit over standard chemotherapy.

- Preclinical and pilot studies also suggest the feasibility of combining cytotoxic chemotherapy with targeted therapy against Bcl-2 overexpression (with Bcl-2 antisense oligonucleotides).

- Preliminary, randomized, phase II data of front-line Pemetrexed (a multi-targeted antifolate) in combination with either cisplatin or carboplatin in ED-SCLC suggest feasibility, with a reasonable toxicity profile.

16

Malignant mesothelioma

Epidemiology

[Robinson BSW, *Lancet* **366**: 397–408, 2005]

- Malignant mesothelioma (MM) is an aggressive but rare malignancy in which cells of the mesothelium become abnormal and divide without control or order.

- Incidence rates have ↑ in the past 20 years.

- 2,000 new cases are diagnosed in the USA each year.

- MM occurs more often in ♂ than in ♀ and risk ↑ with age.

- 80% of cases are believed to derive from occupational or paraoccupational exposure to primary asbestos fiber types; namely crocidolite, amosite, and chrysotile in a ratio of 500:100:1, respectively. [Hodgson JT, *Ann Occup Hyg* **44**: 565–601, 2004].

- The remaining 20% of cases have no clear-cut occupational cause and are believed to be related to etiologic factors, including:
  - Contact with non-industrial fibers such as erionite and exposure to simian virus 40 (SV40).

- SV40, a DNA tumor virus affecting Asian macaques that contaminated poliovirus vaccine stocks used in the late 1950s/early 1960s, has been connected to MM.
  [Carbone M, *Semin Oncol* **29**: 2–17, 2002]
  [Strickler HD, *J Natl Cancer Inst* **85**: 38–45, 2003]

- SV40 appears to inactivate p53 and p-retinoblastoma family proteins, which in turn indirectly affect cyclin-dependent kinase subunits.
  - SV40 also acts synergistically with asbestos to cause malignant transformation of human mesothelial cells.
  [Mossman BT, *Am J Respir Cell Mol Biol* **26**: 167–170, 2002]
  - Data from the SEER (Surveillance, Epidemiology, and End Results) program demonstrated no correlation between pleural mesothelioma incidence rates and poliovirus vaccine exposure for the years 1975–1997.

- Data suggest a critical role for multiple growth factors (e.g. epidermal growth factor, tumor necrosis factor, platelet-derived growth factor, hepatocyte growth factor, and keratinocyte growth factor) in the expansion of transformed mesothelial cell populations via autocrine and paracrine mechanisms.
[Mossman BT, *Am J Respir Cell Mol Biol* **26**: 167–170, 2002]

Prognostic factors

[Herndon JE, *Chest* **113**: 723–731, 1998]
[Curran D, *J Clin Oncol* **16**: 145–152, 1998]

Group	Indicators of poor median survival	Indicators of best median survival
Cancer and Leukemia Group B (CALGB)	Male gender Age > 75 years PS 1 or 2 Pleural disease involvement Chest pain or dyspnea Platelets > 400,000 per µl LDH > 500 IU/l Low hemoglobin	PS 0 Age < 49 years
European Organization for Research and Treatment of Cancer (EORTC)	PS 2 White blood cells > 8300 µl Histologic uncertainty Male gender Sarcomatous histologic subtype	≤ 2 prognostic factors present

PS, performance status.

Osteopontin in malignant mesothelioma

[Pass HI, *N Engl J Med* **353**(15): 1564–1573, 2005]

- Investigated the presence of osteopontin in pleural mesothelioma and determined serum osteopontin levels in three populations: subjects without cancer who were exposed to asbestos, subjects without cancer who were not exposed to asbestos, and patients with pleural mesothelioma who were exposed to asbestos.
  - 69 subjects with asbestos-related non-malignant pulmonary disease were compared with 45 subjects without exposure to asbestos and 76 patients with surgically staged pleural mesothelioma.
  - Tumor tissue was examined for osteopontin using immunohistochemical analysis, and serum osteopontin levels were measured using enzyme-linked immunosorbent assay (ELISA).
  - RESULTS:
    - Serum osteopontin levels in the group with pleural mesothelioma were higher than in the group with exposure to asbestos.
    - Immunohistochemical analysis revealed osteopontin staining of the tumor cells in 36/38 of the samples of pleural mesothelioma.
    - Analysis of the serum osteopontin levels by comparing the receiver operating characteristic (ROC) curve for the group exposed to asbestos with that of the group with mesothelioma had a sensitivity of 77.6% and a specificity of 85.5%, at a cut-off value of 48.3 ng/ml.
    - Subgroup analysis comparing patients with stage I mesothelioma with subjects with exposure to asbestos revealed a sensitivity of 84.6% and a specificity of 88.4%, at a cut-off value of 62.4 ng/ml.
  - CONCLUSION:
    - Serum osteopontin levels can be used to distinguish persons with exposure to asbestos who do not have cancer from those with exposure to asbestos who have pleural mesothelioma.

Role of surgery

[Van Ruth S, *Chest* **123**: 551–561, 2003]
[Jaklitsch MT, *World J Surg* **25**(2): 210–217, 2001]

- Surgery can be diagnostic, palliative, or curative.

- Three surgical procedures have been used for palliative or curative purposes: pleurodesis, pleurectomy with decortication, and extrapleural pneumonectomy.

- No prospective randomized trials comparing these procedures have been done.

- The role of surgery in MM remains controversial.
  [McCormack P, J Thorac Cardiovasc Surg **84**: 834–842, 1982]
  - 149 patients (110 ♂ and 39 ♀) with MM were treated at the Memorial Sloan–Kettering Cancer Center.
  - From 1939–1981.
  - These patients were managed with combined surgical therapy, radiation therapy (XRT), and chemotherapy.
  - RESULTS:
    - No benefit from pulmonary resection was found in the group that had surgical treatment only.
    - Better survival was achieved when the surgery was combined with XRT and chemotherapy.

- [Law MR, Thorax **39**: 255–259, 1984]
  - 150 patients with MM were managed at two hospitals.
  - From 1971–1980.
  - 52 patients received active treatment vs 64 patients who were untreated. Sequential prospective studies of the effect of surgery alone (non-radical parietal pleurectomy and decortication of the lung, removing the bulk of the tumor), chemotherapy (cyclophosphamide, doxorubicin, and vincristine were given for 6 courses), and XRT were performed.
  - RESULTS:
    - There was no significant difference in survival between treatment groups or between treated and untreated patients.

Pleurodesis

- Palliative without cytoreduction.

- May be the procedure of choice for recurrent symptomatic effusions.

- Four agents can be used: talc, tetracycline, doxycycline, and bleomycin.

- There is a possible tumoricidal effect on cell lines, as talc could induce apoptosis in human MM cells.
  [Nasreen N, Am J Respir Crit Care Med **161**: 595–600, 2000]

- Prospective randomized trials of talc vs bleomycin, tetracycline vs bleomycin, and doxycycline vs bleomycin have been done, with equivalent inflammatory reaction and palliation with each agent.
  [Noppen M, Acta Clin Belg **52**: 258–262, 1997]

[Martinez-Moragon E, *Eur Respir J* **10**: 2380–2383, 1997]
[Patz EF Jr, *Chest* **113**: 1305–1311, 1998]

- Mean survival is similar to the length of the natural course of the disease.
  [Canto A, *Thorac Cardiovasc Surg* **45**: 16–19, 1997].

- Failure is associated with mesothelioma with entrapped lung, large solid tumor mass, loculations secondary to multiple thoracenteses, or age > 70 years.

Pleurectomy with decortication

- Involves stripping the pleura from the lung apex to the diaphragm, leaving the lung in place.

- It is more successful than talc pleurodesis.

- Pleurectomy alone has not been shown to prolong survival.

- [Brancatisano RR, *Med J Aust* **154**: 455–457, 1991]
  - Surgical mortality → 1–2%.
  - Median survival → 7–21 months.
  - Effusion control rate → 86–98%.
  - Complications of pleurectomy with decortication:
    – Pneumonia, respiratory insufficiency, empyema, and hemorrhage.
  - Postoperative XRT is limited due to the presence of lung in the radiation field.

Extrapleural pneumonectomy

- Involves the en bloc removal of the parietal and visceral pleura, lung, hemidiaphragm, pericardium, and mediastinal nodes with subsequent reconstruction of the diaphragm and pericardium.

- Classically described for stage I MMs that are technically resectable and encapsulated by the parietal pleura.

- Technically complex and associated with significant perioperative morbidity and mortality, with 60% overall incidence of complications.
  [Sugarbaker DJ, *J Thorac Cardiovasc Surg* **128**: 138–146, 2004]

- Limited to skilled surgeons and to the few patients who are candidates for it.
  [Grodin SC, *Chest* **116**: 450S, 1999]

- [Aisner J, *Chest* **107**: 332S–344S, 1995]
  - The only procedure possible when a thick tumor rind obliterates the pleural space.
  - Surgical mortality → 5–31%.
  - Median survival → 4–21 months.
  - Complications of extrapleural pneumonectomy (EPP):
    - Bronchial leaks, empyema, vocal cord paralysis, chylothorax, patch failure, arrhythmias, and respiratory insufficiency.
- [Rusch VW, *J Thorac Cardiovasc Surg* **102**: 1–9, 1991]
  - 83 patients with untreated MM.
  - Prospective multi-institutional trial.
  - From 1985 to 1988.
  - 20 patients underwent extrapleural pneumonectomy, and the remaining 63 patients had more limited surgery with or without adjuvant therapy or had non-surgical treatment.
  - RESULTS:
    - Recurrence-free survival was significantly longer for patients undergoing EPP than for the other two groups, but there was no difference in overall survival between the three groups.
    - EPP was associated with ↑ likelihood of relapse in distant sites than were limited operation and non-surgical treatment.
- EPP alone does not influence survival. However, it is an excellent means of symptoms palliation.
  [Rusch VW, *J Thorac Cardiovasc Surg* **111**: 815–825, 1996]

Radiotherapy

[Ahamad A, *Int J Radiat Oncol Biol Phys* **55**: 768–775, 2003]

- The role of XRT is limited because of the involvement of the diffuse pleural surface and the interlobular fissures, and the radiation sensitivity of the surrounding organs.

- XRT may play a role in preventing recurrences in the chest wall after thoracoscopy/thoracotomy and after pleurectomy or EPP.

- There are no randomized trials demonstrating the efficacy of XRT.

- It can provide local palliation in up to 50% of patients.
  [De Graaf-Strukowska L, *Int J Radiat Oncol Biol Phys* **43**: 511–516, 1999]

- Various methods have been used, but the most successful is intensity-modulated XRT.

Photodynamic therapy

[Hahn SM, *Curr Treat Options Oncol* **2**(5): 375–383, 2002]

- Photodynamic therapy (PDT) is a light-based cancer treatment that requires the use of a photosensitizing agent and light of a wavelength specific to the absorption characteristics of the sensitizer in the presence of oxygen.

- The treatment effect of PDT is superficial, mostly because of the limited depth of light absorption by the tissues.

- Theoretically, PDT is an ideal treatment for tissue surfaces and body cavities after surgical debulking procedures.

- It can be used to treat the lung surface after a pleurectomy; and therefore patients may be treated with a pleurectomy rather than with EPP.

- There is no convincing proof that the use of PDT is superior to the use of other adjuvant therapies or to surgery alone.

Chemotherapy for mesothelioma

Single agents

[Ong ST, *J Clin Oncol* **14**: 1007–1017, 1996]
[Berghmas T, *Lung Cancer* **38**: 111–121, 2002]
[Tomek S, *Br J Cancer* **88**: 167–174, 2003]

- Platinum agents (cisplatin and carboplatin), anthracyclines (doxorubicin, detorubicin, and pirarubicin), and antimetabolites (methotrexate, gemcitabine, and Pemetrexed).

- Symptomatic improvement → 15–20%.

- Median survival → 7–9 months.

Combination regimens

- *Cisplatin + doxorubicin.*
  [Henss H, *Onkologie* **11**: 118–120, 1988]
  [Ardizzoni A, *Cancer* **67**: 2984–2987, 1991]
  [Chahinian AP, *J Clin Oncol* **11**: 1559–1565, 1993]
  - Three phase II trials.
  - Total 78 patients.

- RESULTS:
  - Response rate → 14–42%.
  - Median survival → 7–12 months.
- *Cisplatin + flurouracil + mytomycin + etoposide.*
  [Kasseyet S, *Cancer* **85**(8): 1740–1749, 1999]
  - Phase II trial.
  - 45 patients.
  - RESULTS:
    - Partial response → 38%.
    - Median response duration → 12 months.
- *Cisplatin + gemcitabine.*
  [Byrne MJ, *J Clin Oncol* **17**(1): 25–30, 1999]
  - Phase II trial.
  - 21 patients.
  - RESULTS:
    - Partial response → 48%.
    - Symptomatic improvement in 90% of patients.
    - Median response duration → 6.2 months.
- *Cisplatin + Pemetrexed.*
  [Vogelzang NJ, *J Clin Oncol* **21**: 2636–2644, 2003]
  - Single-blinded, phase II, prospective randomized trial.
  - 456 patients.
  - RESULTS:
    - Combination was superior to cisplatin alone.
    - Response rate → 41% vs 17%.
    - Median survival → 12.1 vs 9.3 months.
    - These differences were more evident in the group of patients receiving folic acid and vitamin B_{12} supplementation.
    - Overall survival predictors: performance status, disease stage, histologic subtype, white blood cell count, vitamin supplementation, and cystathionine levels.
  - CONCLUSION:
    - Cisplatin + Pemetrexed: standard first-line regimen.
- *Carboplatin + Pemetrexed.*
  [Hughes A, *J Clin Oncol* **20**: 3533–3544, 2002]
  - Phase I trial.
  - 25 patients.
  - RESULTS:
    - Response rate → 32%.
    - Symptomatic improvement in 70% of patients.

- *Cisplatin + raltitrexed.*
  [Van Meerbeeck JP, *J Clin Oncol* **23**: 6881–6889, 2005]
  - Phase III trial.
  - 250 patients.
  - Cisplatin vs cisplatin + raltitrexed.
  - RESULTS:
    – Combination was superior.
    – Response rate → 23.6% vs 14%.
    – Median survival → 11.4 vs 8.8 months.
    – 1-year survival → 46% vs 40%.
    – No toxic deaths seen.
  - CONCLUSION:
    – The combination improves survival and is superior to cisplatin alone.

- *Oxaliplatin + raltitrexed.*
  [Fizazi K, *J Clin Oncol* **21**(2): 349–354, 2003]
  - Phase II.
  - 70 patients (including 15 pretreated).
  - RESULTS:
    – Partial response → 20%.
    – Symptomatic response → 30–36%.
    – 1-year survival rate → 26%.
    – Median survival → 11 months for non-pretreated patients and 7.8% for pretreated patients.

- *Oxaliplatin + gemcitabine.*
  [Schutte W, *Clin Lung Cancer* **4**(5): 294–297, 2003]
  - Multicenter, phase II trial.
  - 25 patients.
  - RESULTS:
    – Partial response → 40%.
    – Median survival → 13 months.

New agents

- ZD0473.
  [Giaccone G, *Eur J Cancer* **38**(Suppl 8): S19, 2002]
  - Oral cisplatin analogue.
  - 47 patients.
  - 83% previously treated with cisplatin.
  - RESULTS:
    – 5 minor responses.
    – Median survival → 203 days.

17

Lung cancer in the elderly population and poor performance status

[Gridelli C, *Chest* **128**(2): 947–957, 2005]
[Gridelli C, *J Clin Oncol* **23**: 3125–3137]
[Govindan R, *Semin Oncol* **31**(Suppl 11): 27–31, 2004]

- The population of the USA is aging, and the proportion of the population that will be > 65 years old by 2030 is expected to be > 20%.

- > 50% of cases of advanced non-small-cell lung cancer (NSCLC) are diagnosed in people aged ≥ 65 years and 35–40% are diagnosed in people > 70 years old.
  - In most trials, on average, only 20% of participants are > 70 years old.

- In general, 'elderly' is defined with regard to lung cancer as age > 70 years old.

- Surveillance, Epidemiology, and End Results (SEER) data in the USA from the 1990s suggest that 69 years is the median age of diagnosis for lung cancer.
  - Cancer risk increases with increasing age.
  - With the aging population the prevalence of lung cancer in the elderly is expected to increase.

Age as a prognostic factor

[Stanley KE, *J Natl Cancer Inst* **65**: 25–32, 1980]

- An analysis was done of the role of 77 variables in the prognosis of lung cancer. <u>Age showed no impact on survival</u>.

- The most important prognostic factors were performance status (PS), extent of disease, and weight loss over the preceding 6 months.

- There are several options for the treatment of elderly patients:
  - Best supportive care without chemotherapy.
  - Single-agent chemotherapy (usually with a third-generation drug).
  - Non-platinum-based combination chemotherapy.
  - Platinum-based combination chemotherapy.
  - New biological agents.

- As people age there is a progressive decline in the functional reserve of multiple organ systems. However, as people age differently, each patient should undergo a comprehensive assessment, and the benefits vs the risks of chemotherapy should be assessed individually.

Guidelines from the National Comprehensive Cancer Network

1. Geriatric assessment for individuals aged ≥ 70 years.
2. Dose adjustment of chemotherapy to the renal function for patients aged ≥ 65 years.
3. Prophylactic use of filgrastim or pegfilgrastim in patients aged ≥ 65 years receiving chemotherapy of a dose intensity comparable to that of cyclophosphamide, doxorubicin, vincristine, and prednisone.
4. Maintenance of hemoglobin levels at > 12 g/dl.
5. Preferential use of chemotherapy of low toxicity.

Best supportive care vs single-agent chemotherapy

- Several trials have compared whether to give chemotherapy to elderly patients. The general conclusion is that chemotherapy is beneficial.

- Elderly Lung Cancer Vinorelbine Italian Study (ELVIS) trial.
  [The ELVIS Group, *J Natl Cancer Inst* **91**: 66–72, 1999]
  Randomized, phase III study of the effect of vinorelbine on quality of life (QOL) and survival in elderly patients with advanced NSCLC.
  - 161 patients aged > 70 years.
  - Randomly assigned to receive best supportive care or chemotherapy (vinorelbine 30 mg/m^2 on days 1 and 8 q 3 weeks for a maximum of 6 cycles).
  - Main endpoint: QOL (assessed using European Organization for Research and Treatment of Cancer core questionnaire (QLQ-C30) and lung-cancer-specific module (QLQ-LC13)).

- RESULTS:
  - Chemotherapy group had significantly longer survival (28 vs 21 weeks; log-rank test, $p = 0.03$), and a greater chance of 6-month survival (55% vs 41%) and 1-year survival (32% vs 14%).
  - With regard to QOL, those receiving vinorelbine scored better than controls on global health status, several functional scales (cognitive, social, physical), fatigue, pain, dyspnea and cough.

Group	No. of patients	OR (%)	Median survival (months)	1-year overall survival (%)
Vinorelbine	78	20	6.5	32
Best supportive care	76	–	4.9	14

Single-agent chemotherapy (usually with a third-generation drug) vs combination therapy

- Several drugs, including vinorelbine, oral vinorelbine, gemcitabine, paclitaxel, and docetaxel, have been tested for use in elderly patients with NSCLC.

- Currently the favored approach for elderly patients is single-agent chemotherapy sequentially.
  - In an effort to ↓ the negative effects of chemotherapy.
  - But trials are conflicting, with some suggesting a trend to increased survival with combination chemotherapy upfront.
  - Therefore, again, each patient should be assessed individually.

- Southwest Oncology Group (SWOG) (S0027).

Sequential therapy

- [Hesketh PJ, *Proc Am Soc Oncol* 23: 627 (abstract 7056), 2004]
  - Phase II trial.
  - For 75 elderly patients with PS 0 or 1.
  - Sequential vinorelbine and docetaxel in patients with advanced NSCLC aged > 70 years or with PS 2.
  - RESULTS:
    - Response rate 21%; median survival 9 months; good tolerability.

Combination therapy vs single-agent therapy

Non-platinum combination treatment in elderly patients with NSCLC

- Southern Italy Cooperative Group (SICOG) trial.
  [Frasci G, *Lung Cancer* **34**(Suppl): S65–S69, 2001]
  - Gemcitabine + vinorelbine vs vinorelbine alone in patients with NSCLC.
  - Age ≥ 70 years at diagnosis.
  - Randomized to vinorelbine 30 mg/m² on days 1 and 8 q 3 weeks vs vinorelbine 30 mg/m² on days 1 and 8 + gemcitabine 1250 mg/m² on days 1 and 8 q 3 weeks.
  - RESULTS:

Regimen	No. of patients	Overall response rate (%)	Median survival (months)
Vinorelbine	60	15	4.2
Vinorelbine + gemcitabine	60	22	6.7

  - Although there is significant survival ($p < 0.01$) and a better response rate for the combination, the 18 week survival for vinorelbine is lower than previous trials.
  - CONCLUSION:
    - Gemcitabine + vinorelbine yields better survival outcome than vinorelbine alone in elderly patients with advanced NSCLC.

- Multicenter Italian Lung Cancer in the Elderly Study (MILES) trial.
  [Gridelli C, *J Natl Cancer Inst* **95**: 362–372, 2003]
  - Chemotherapy for elderly patients with advanced NSCLC.
  - Randomized, phase III trial.
  - Patients aged ≥ 70 years.
  - Vinorelbine 30 mg/m² vs gemcitabine 1200 mg/m² vs vinorelbine 25 mg/m² + gemcitabine 1000 mg/m².
  - RESULTS:

Regimen	No. of patients	Overall response rate (%)	Median survival (months)
Vinorelbine	233	18	8.3
Gemcitabine	233	16	6.5
Vinorelbine + gemcitabine	232	21	6.9

- CONCLUSION:
  - Single-agent therapy with either gemcitabine or vinorelbine is preferable to combination treatment of advanced NSCLC in elderly patients.
- Combination treatment with weekly docetaxel + gemcitabine for advanced NSCLC in elderly patients and patients with poor performance status.
  [Hainsworth JD, *Clin Lung Cancer* 5: 33–38, 2003]
  - Minnie Pearl Cancer Research Network, phase II trial.
  - 64 patients (aged ≥ 70 years) with poor PS.
  - Docetaxel 30 mg/m² + gemcitabine 800 mg/m² on days 1, 8 and 15 of each 28-day cycle.
  - RESULTS:
    - 28% response; median survival 7.0 months.

Platinum-based combination therapy in elderly patients with non-small-cell lung cancer

- [Rinaldi M, *Ann Oncol* 5 (Suppl 8): 58 (abstract 0289), 1994]
  A retrospective analysis of cisplatin-based chemotherapy in elderly patients with NSCLC.
  - RESULTS:
    - Significant increase in death with increasing age within 30 days of starting chemotherapy (0.5%, 3.3%, 3.2%, 7.1%, and 12.5%, for patients aged ≤ 54, 55–59, 60–64, 65–69, and ≥ 70 years, respectively; $p = 0.0001$).
    - See Table 17.1.
- Several trials have been conducted substituting carboplatin for cisplatin, due to the lower rates of nausea/vomiting, neuropathy, nephrotoxicity, and neurotoxicity with carboplatin.
  - See Table 17.2.
- Due to no current, elderly-specific, prospective, phase III trials of platinum-based therapy in NSCLC, a number of retrospective subset analysis have been done.
- Eastern Cooperative Oncology Group (ECOG) 5592.
  [Langer CJ, *J Natl Cancer Inst* 94 (3): 173–181, 2002]
  - Randomization to cisplatin 75 mg/m² +:
    - Etoposide 100 mg/m² on days 1–3.
    - Paclitaxel 135 mg/m²/24 hours on day 2.

Table 17.1 Phase II trials with a cisplatin-based chemotherapy regimen

Regimen	Age (years)	No. of patients	ORR (%)	MS (months)
Cisplatin 60–90 mg/m² + vinorelbine 25 mg/m² [a]	> 70	44	54	7.2
Cisplatin 50 mg/m² q 3 weeks + gemcitabine 1000 mg/m² [b]	≥ 70	46	35	10.2
Cisplatin 35 mg/m² weekly + gemcitabine 1000 mg/m² [c]	≥ 68	15	40	9
Cisplatin 35 mg/m² weekly + gemcitabine 1000 mg/m² [d]	≥ 70	48	31.8	9
Cisplatin 25 mg/m² weekly + docetaxel 20 mg/m² [e]	≥ 75	33	52	15.8

MS, median survival; ORR, overall response rate.
[a][Martins SJ, *BMC Cancer* **4**: 69, 2004]
[b][Feliu J, *Cancer Chemother Pharmacol* **52**(3): 247–252, 2003]
[c][Lippe P, *Minerva Med* **91**: 53–57, 2000]
[d][Berardi R, *Oncology* **65**:198–203, 2003]
[e][Ohe Y, *Ann Oncol* **15**: 45–50, 2004]

- – Paclitaxel 250 mg/m²/24 hours on day 2 + granulocyte colony-stimulating factor (GCSF).
- Breakdown by 'elderly' (age ≥ 70 years) vs 'young' (< 70 years).
  - – The elderly group had increased cardiovascular ($p = 0.0089$) and respiratory ($p = 0.0441$) comorbidities.
  - – The elderly group showed increased leukopenia ($p = 0.0001$) and neuropsychological toxicity ($p = 0.0025$).
  - – No difference in baseline QOL, time to progression, or median survival.
  - – Conclusion: PS is a greater predictor of survival than age.
- ECOG 1594
  [Langer CJ, *J Natl Cancer Inst* **94**: 173–181, 2002]
  [Langer CJ, *Proc Am Soc Clin Oncol* **22**: 639 (abstract), 2003]
  [Schiller JH, *N Engl J Med* **346**: 92–98, 2002]
  - Data analyzed by Langer and Schiller.

Table 17.2 Phase II trials with a carboplatin-based chemotherapy regimen

Regimen	Age (years)	No. of patients	ORR (%)	MS (months)
Carboplatin + vinorelbine[a]	≥ 70	22	14	NR
Carboplatin + vinorelbine[b]	≥ 60	44	27	6.5
Carboplatin + gemcitabine[c]	≥ 65	88	37.5	9.0
Carboplatin + paclitaxel[d]	≥ 70	50	16	7.1
Carboplatin + paclitaxel[e]	≥ 70	25	36	NR
Carboplatin + paclitaxel[f]	≥ 65	35	40	8.6
Carboplatin + paclitaxel[g]	≥ 70	25	25	11.3

MS, median survival; NR, not recorded; ORR, overall response rate.
[a][Colleoni M, Sixth International Congress on Anti-Cancer Treatment, Paris, France, Feb 6–9, 1996]
[b][Santomaggio CR, *J Chemother* **8**(Suppl): 104, 1996]
[c][Maestu I, *Lung Cancer* **42**: 345–354, 2003]
[d][Marland T, *Proc Am Soc Clin Oncol* **20**: 267b, 2001]
[e][Molinier O, *Proc Am Soc Clin Oncol* **22**: 693 (abstract 2786), 2003]
[f][Okamoto I, *Proc Am Soc Clin Oncol* **23**: 672 (abstract 7237), 2004]
[g][Hensing TA, *Cancer* **98**: 779–788, 2003]

- Four drug combinations (cisplatin + paclitaxel, cisplatin + docetaxel, cisplatin + gemcitabine, and carboplatin + paclitaxel) were evaluated as first-line therapy for NSCLC.
- RESULTS:
  - No significant differences were reported for response rates (24.5% vs 22.1%) or median survival (8.3 vs 8.2 months) for the 227 (20%) patients aged ≥ 70 years compared with those aged < 70 years.
  - Marginally significant ($p = 0.04$) increase in grade 4 toxicities.
- SWOG 9509/9308.
  [Kelly K, *Proc Am Soc Clin Oncol* **20**: 329a (abstract), 2001]
  - SWOG 9509 compared carboplatin + paclitaxel with cisplatin + vinorelbine.
  - SWOG 9308 compared cisplatin + vinorelbine with cisplatin alone.
    - Subset analysis of 117 of the 608 evaluable patients.

- No statistically significant influence of age on survival (8.6 vs 6.9 months for those aged < 70 years vs those aged ≥ 70 years; $p = 0.06$), time to progression (4.2 vs 3.9 months; $p = 0.62$), or toxicity.

- Carboplatin + paclitaxel ×4 cycles vs carboplatin + paclitaxel until progression.
  [Hensing TA, *Cancer* **98**: 779–788, 2003]
  - 67 patients aged ≥ 70 years, 163 patients aged < 70 years.
  - RESULTS:
    - There was no difference in overall response rate (27% vs 20% for those aged ≥ 70 years and < 70 years, respectively) or median survival (7.1 vs 7.8 months for those aged ≥ 70 years and < 70 years, respectively).

- TAX 326.
  [Fossella F, *Proc Am Soc Clin Oncol* **22**: 629 (abstract), 2003]
  - A subset analysis of 401 patients aged ≥ 65 years, comparing cisplatin + docetaxel with carboplatin + docetaxel and cisplatin + vinorelbine.
  - RESULTS:
    - Median survival 12.6 months vs carboplatin + docetaxel (9.0 months) vs cisplatin + vinorelbine (9.9 months).
    - No increase in toxicity in the elderly population, with those receiving carboplatin + docetaxel showing the least toxicity.

- The Cancer and Leukemia Group B (CALGB) 9730.
  [Lilenbaum R, *J Clin Oncol* **23**: 190–196, 2005]
  - Single-agent vs combination chemotherapy in advanced NSCLC.
  - Paclitaxel 225 mg/m² on day 1 q 3 weeks vs paclitaxel 225 mg/m² on day 1 q 3 weeks + carboplatin AUC = 6 on day 1 q 3 weeks for a maximum of 6 cycles.
  - RESULTS:

Regimen	Age (years)	No. of patients	Overall response rate (%)	Median survival (months)
Paclitaxel	> 70	78	21	5.8
Paclitaxel	< 70	199	15	6.8
Paclitaxel + carboplatin	> 70	77	36	8.0
Paclitaxel + carboplatin	< 70	207	28	9.0

- CONCLUSIONS:
  - Elderly patients have a similar overall response rate and survival to younger patients. Combination chemotherapy showed a trend to improvement in survival, but this trend was not significant.

Targeted therapy

- Gefitinib (Iressa) and erlotinib (Tarceva) are two inhibitors of epidermal growth factor receptor tyrosine kinase that have demonstrated activity in heavily pretreated patients with NSCLC.

- They are generally well tolerated with mild adverse events, except for a rash.

- Currently gefitinib is not approved in the USA except for patients already on the drug and responding.

- Erlotinib.
  [Johnson BE, *Proc Am Soc Clin Oncol* **23**: 633 (abstract), 2004]
  36 patients aged ≥ 70 years had an overall response rate of 13.2%, with 50% showing stable disease. Median survival times have not been reported.

- Several trials of Pemetrexed in elderly patients are ongoing in the USA and Europe, but the data have not yet been published.

Poor performance status in NSCLC

- Several trials (see below) have shown that patients with a PS of 2 or worse have shorter survival.

- ECOG 1581 showed that a PS of 2 had no objective responses, a median survival of 10 weeks, and 10% toxic deaths vs 2–3% of deaths for patients with a PS of 0 or 1.

- Hellenic Cooperative Group Efforts.
  [Kosimidis J, *Ann Oncol* **11**: 799–805, 2000]
  [Kosimidis J, *Clin Oncol* **20**: 3578–3585, 2002]
  - Two separate phase III trials.
  - Carboplatin (AUC = 6) + paclitaxel (225 vs 175 mg/m^2).
  - Paclitaxel + carboplatin vs paclitaxel + gemcitabine: the time to progression and median survival were shorter in patients with a PS of 2.

- RESULTS:

Performance status	Time to progression (months)	Median survival (months)	1-year overall survival (%)
Carboplatin (AUC = 6) + paclitaxel (225 vs 175 mg/m²)			
0–1	6.3	11.25	NA
2	2.4	3.8	NA
Paclitaxel + carboplatin vs paclitaxel + gemcitabine			
0–1	6.6	11.1	44.4
2	3.8	5.9	20

NA, not available.

- ECOG 1594.
  [Sweeney CJ, *Cancer* **92**: 2639–2647, 2001]
  - In a subset analysis of PS 2 patients (68/1207 patients) the median survival was only 4.1 months.

- CALGB 9730.
  [Lilenbaum R, *J Clin Oncol* **23**: 190–196, 2005]
  - Single agent vs combination chemotherapy in advanced NSCLC.
  - RESULTS:

Regimen	Performance status	No. of patients	Overall response rate (%)	Median survival (months)
Paclitaxel	2	50	10	2.4
Paclitaxel	0–1	227	19	7.8
Paclitaxel + carboplatin	2	49	24	4.7
Paclitaxel + carboplatin	0–1	235	26	9.5

- CONCLUSIONS:
  - This trial confirmed that patients with poor performance had shorter survival, but in this trial combination therapy was better than single-agent chemotherapy.
- For all patients with a PS of 2 the treatment toxicities should be weighed carefully against the benefits, and alternative approaches should be considered.

- Use new active single agents.
- Use schedules with favorable toxicity profiles.
- Use agents sequentially.
- Avoid cisplatin.
- Enrol the patient in a clinical trial.

Take-home messages: elderly vs 'poor risk' patients with advanced non-small-cell lung cancer

1. Elderly vs 'poor risk' patients with advanced NSCLC.

2. 'Healthy' elderly fare as well on standard chemotherapy approaches as younger patients.

3. 'Poor risk' patients (PS 2, low albumin, weight loss) fare poorly.

4. Consider alternative approaches.

18

Targeted therapy in non-small-cell lung cancer

Introduction

[Schiller J, *Semin Respir Crit Care Med* **25**(Suppl 1): 11–16, 2004]
[Morrow P, *Semin Respir Crit Care Med* **26**: 323–332, 2005]

- The success of targeted therapy in other malignant diseases such as chronic myelogenous leukemia and gastrointestinal stromal tumors has also been recently recognized in non-small-cell lung cancer (NSCLC).
  - Targeting certain lung tumor cell receptors has resulted in progression-free and overall survival (OS) advantage.

- Several classes of compounds now target specific steps in cellular proliferation and apoptosis.
  - These include epidermal growth factor receptor (EGFR) inhibitors, vascular endothelial growth factor (VEGF) antibodies, matrix metalloproteinase inhibitors, farnesyltransferase inhibitors, retinoids, proteosome inhibitors, raf/MAPK (mitogen-activated protein kinase) inhibitors, and others.

- Although many of these agents have shown promise in NSCLC, a cautious perspective must be maintained, because agents such as bexarotene (retinoid), which showed promise in early studies, have proved disappointing in randomized trials.

- As the number of therapeutic agents ↑ in NSCLC, there will be greater emphasis on the selection of an appropriate patient population in which to give specific, targeted therapies.
[Blumenschein G, *Proc Am Soc Clin Oncol* **23**: 621 (abstract 7001), 2005]

Approved compounds for non-small-cell lung cancer and mechanism of action

- Gefitinib (Iressa): an EGFR inhibitor.
- Erlotinib (Tarceva): an EGFR inhibitor.

Epidermal growth factor receptor

[Schlessinger J, *Cell* **103**: 211–225, 2000]

- The epidermal growth factor (EGF) family of receptors share a common molecular structure, which has a carboxyl-terminal intracellular domain that has a tyrosine kinase (TK) activity.
- Binding of ligands to the amino-terminal extracellular domain of the EGFR activates the receptor and its signaling pathway.
  - This induces a cascade of intracellular modulation and activation of processes that regulate differentiation, proliferation, migration, and survival. Such signaling pathways induced by EGFR are MAPK which regulates gene transcription and proliferation, and PI3K, which mediates cell survival.

Gefitinib

- Gefitinib (Iressa) is the first targeted therapy approved for NSCLC.
  - It reversibly inhibits HER1 TK.
- A phase I trial showed the efficacy of gefitinib when used as a single agent in heavily pretreated NSCLC patients.
- Dose: 250 mg/day p.o.
  - May be taken long term.
- Half-life → 28 hours and oral bioavailability → 59%.
- Side-effects are usually dose-dependent skin reaction and diarrhea (which represent the dose-limiting toxicities).
- Iressa NSCLC Trial Assessing Combination Trials (INTACT).
  [Giaccone G, *J Clin Oncol* **22**: 777–784, 2004]
  [Herbst R, *J Clin Oncol* **22**: 785–794, 2004]
  - Two large, randomized, placebo-controlled, phase III trials named INTACT-1 (gemcitabine + cisplatin) and INTACT-2 (paclitaxel +

carboplatin) showed that gefitinib does <u>not</u> add additional thera-peutic benefit over single-agent chemotherapy.
- The results of INTACT-2 showed a trend of a possible main-tenance effect of gefitinib in patients with NSCLC who responded to chemotherapy, suggesting a role for sequencing and mainten-ance therapy.

- Molecular markers in gefitinib trials: Iressa Dose Evaluation in Advanced Lung Cancer (IDEAL) and Iressa NSCLC Trial Assessing Combination Treatment (INTACT).
[Bell DW, *J Clin Oncol* **23**(31): 8081–8092, 2005]
  - Analyzed the incidence of EGFR mutation and gene amplification from patients with NSCLC enrolled into IDEAL and INTACT.
  - IDEAL-1 and IDEAL-2 trials: involved gefitinib monotherapy (250 or 500 mg/day) in 425 previously treated patients with advanced NSCLC.
  - INTACT-1 and INTACT-2 trials: compared chemotherapy vs chemotherapy + gefitinib (250 or 500 mg/day, respectively) in 2,130 previously untreated NSCLC patients.
  - Paraffin-embedded diagnostic tumor blocks were available from 643 patients for EGFR gene sequence and amplification (from the IDEAL trials 119 tumor samples were retrieved and from the INTACT trials 524 samples were available).
  - RESULTS:
    - EGFR mutations correlated with clinical features of gefitinib response: adenocarcinoma histology, non-smoker, ♀, and Asian ethnicity.
    - This correlation was not seen in patients whose tumors had EGFR amplification.
    - IDEAL trials: 6/13 (46%) tumors were positive for EGFR, 2/7 with gene amplification, and 5/56 with neither mutation nor amplification responded to gefitinib ($p = 0.001$ for either EGFR mutation or amplification vs neither abnormality).
    - INTACT trials: no correlation was found between EGFR geno-type and response to chemotherapy + gefitinib.
  - CONCLUSIONS:
    - These molecular analyses identified distinct subsets of NSCLC with ↑ response to gefitinib.
    - The combined therapy (gefitinib + chemotherapy) did <u>not</u> improve the survival in patients with positive EGFR mutation and gene amplification.
  - LIMITATION OF THE STUDY:
    - Retrospective analysis.

- Iressa Survival Evaluation in Lung Cancer (ISEL).
  [Thatcher N, *Lancet* **366**: 1527–1537, 2005]
  - Phase III, randomized trial.
  - 1,692 lung cancer patients.
  - RESULTS:
    - Gefitinib failed to significantly prolong survival vs placebo in the overall population (hazard ratio (HR) 0.89, $p = 0.11$, median survival 5.6 vs 5.1 months), or in patients with adenocarcinoma (HR 0.83, $p = 0.07$, median survival 6.3 vs 5.4 months).
    - There was a statistically significant improvement in tumor shrinkage (objective response rate), which did not translate into a statistically significant survival benefit.
    - Subsets of the patient population in these studies, including Asians and never-smokers, did experience significant clinical improvement and provided a basis for further studies.
    - Gefitinib is currently indicated only for NSCLC patients who have already received benefit from gefitinib.
  - CONCLUSION:
    - Approval of gefitinib was recently withdrawn. Gefitinib monotherapy failed to demonstrate a significant survival benefit compared with placebo.

Erlotinib

- Erlotinib (Tarceva) causes a reversible inhibition of HER1 TK.

- Half-life → 24.4 hours at a dose of 150 mg/day p.o.

- Major side-effect → acneiform rash.

- [Herbst RS, *Semin Oncol* **30**(3 Suppl): 34–46, 2003]
  - Phase II trial.
  - 56 patients who failed platinum-based chemotherapy and had > 10% EGFR (+) cells.
  - RESULTS:
    - Response rate → 12%.
    - Prolonged stable disease → 39%.

- [Giaccone G, *Proc Am Soc Clin Oncol* **23**: 638 (abstract 7073), 2005]
  - A phase II trial that evaluated the efficacy and safety of first-line erlotinib in patients with advanced NSCLC.
  - 54 untreated patients (53 assessable) with stage IIIB/IV NSCLC and performance status (PS) 0–2 were enrolled to receive erlotinib 150 mg/day until disease progression or withdrawal.

- Endpoint: rate of non-progression in > 50% of patients after 6 weeks of treatment.
- Secondary endpoints: objective response, disease control rate, duration of response, time to progression, survival, and safety.
- RESULTS:
  - Non-progression rate → 55%.
  - Best response was: 1 complete response (CR), 12 partial response (PR), 16 stable disease, 17 progression of disease, 7 not evaluable (RR 24.5%; 95% CI, 13.8–38.3).
  - Up to May 2005, 14 patients had not progressed and 12 had been treated for 6 months or longer.
  - Responses were observed in ♂ (1 CR, 3 PR) and ♀ (9 PR), mostly in adenocarcinoma (7) and in bronchioalveolar carcinoma (BAC) (4), in non- or former smokers (12).
  - Erlotinib was found to be active and well tolerated as first-line monotherapy in advanced NSCLC.

- Tarceva Responses in Conjunction with Paclitaxel and Carboplatin (TRIBUTE) and Tarceva Lung Cancer Investigation (TALENT) trials. [Gatzemeier U, *Proc Am Soc Clin Oncol* **23**: 617 (abstract 7010), 2004] [Herbst R, Proc Am Soc Clin Oncol 23: **617** (abstract 7011), 2004]
  - Two large, randomized trials of the combination of chemotherapy with or without erlotinib in untreated patients diagnosed with NSCLC.
  - These studies, TRIBUTE (carboplatin + paclitaxel ± erlotinib) and TALENT (cisplatin + gemcitabine ± erlotinib) showed that erlotinib did <u>not</u> confer survival advantage over chemotherapy alone.

- TRIBUTE trial.
  [Herbst RS, *J Clin Oncol* **23**: 5892–5999, 2005]
  - Phase III, randomized trial; untreated patients with advanced (stage IIIB/IV) NSCLC and good PS.
  - Carboplatin + paclitaxel ± erlotinib 150 mg/day vs placebo (6 cycles of therapy), followed by maintenance therapy with erlotinib.
  - 1,079 patients were enrolled (539 erlotinib, 540 placebo). 1,059 patients were assessable (526 erlotinib, 533 placebo).
  - RESULTS:
    - Median survival: 10.6 vs 10.5 months for erlotinib and placebo, respectively ($p = 0.95$).
    - No difference was found for overall response or time to progression (TTP).
    - Non-smokers (72 erlotinib, 44 placebo) had an improved OS in the erlotinib group (22.5 vs 10.1 months).

- No other prespecified factors showed an impact on OS with erlotinib therapy.
  - CONCLUSION:
    - There is no survival advantage between chemotherapy alone or in combination with erlotinib in previously untreated NSCLC.
- BR.21 trial.
  [Shepherd F, N Engl J Med **253**: 123–132, 2005]
  - A multicenter, randomized, placebo-controlled study from the National Cancer Institute of Canada.
  - RESULTS:
    - Showed for the first time that single-agent erlotinib prolonged survival in patients after first- or second-line therapy.
    - The overall response rate (ORR) was 8.9% and OS was 6.7 months for erlotinib and 4.7 months for placebo ($p < 0.001$).

- Retrospective studies of erlotinib and gefitinib found never-smoker, ♀, East Asian ethnicity, adenocarcinoma histologic type, and EGFR mutations in exons 18–21 to be factors associated with a better response rate.
  [Kris M, JAMA **290**: 2149–2158, 2003]
  [Fukuoka M, J Clin Oncol **21**: 2237–2246, 2003]
  [Pao W, J Clin Oncol **23**: 2556–2568, 2005]
  [Shepherd F, N Engl J Med **253**: 123–132, 2005]

- Molecular markers in erlotinib trials.
  [Eberhard DA, J Clin Oncol **23**: 5900–5909, 2005]
  - Studied EGFR as well as K-ras mutation status in patients treated with chemotherapy alone or in combination with erlotinib.
  - EGFR exons 18–21 and K-ras exon 2 were sequenced in tumors from 274 patients who participated in the phase III, TRIBUTE trial and who were randomly assigned to carboplatin + paclitaxel with erlotinib or placebo.
  - Survival, response rate, and TTP were analyzed.
  - RESULTS:
    - EGFR was detected in 13% of the tumors.
    - Irrespective of the treatment received, EGFR mutation was associated with longer survival ($p < 0.001$).
    - Those who received erlotinib had an improved response rate ($p < 0.05$) and a better TTP ($p = 0.092$), but not improved survival ($p = 0.96$).
    - The K-ras mutation was found in 21% of patients.
    - Patients who received erlotinib and had a (+) K-ras mutation showed a significantly ↓ TTP and OS.

- CONCLUSIONS:
  - The presence of the EGFR mutation may predict a better outcome in patients with advanced NSCLC treated with chemotherapy ± erlotinib.
  - The presence of the *K-ras* mutation seems to confer a poor clinical outcome for NSCLC patients when treated with chemotherapy and erlotinib.
- LIMITATION OF THE STUDY:
  - Retrospective analysis.

Where are we going with the molecular markers for tyrosine kinase inhibitors?

- ↑ EGFR gene copy number was associated with improved survival in NSCLC and advanced BAC patients treated with gefitinib monotherapy.
  [Cappuzzo F, *J Natl Cancer Inst* **97**: 643–655, 2005]
  [Hirsch FR, *J Clin Oncol* **23**: 6838–6845, 2005]

- However, such an association did not exist for a combination of gefitinib + chemotherapy in NSCLC.
  [Bell DW, *J Clin Oncol* **23**: 8081–8092, 2005]

- Amplification of the *HER2* gene was also associated with gefitinib activity in NSCLC.
  [Cappuzzo F, *J Clin Oncol* **23**: 5007–5018, 2005]

- The BR.21 study also failed to demonstrate any association between EGFR gene copy number and survival in NSCLC patients treated with single-agent erlotinib.
  [Tsao MS, *N Engl J Med* **353**: 133–144, 2005]

- In conclusion, the true correlation between EGFR/HER gene amplification and sensitivity to different EGFR-targeted therapies remains an important focus of clinical investigation.

Compounds in clinical development for therapy for non-small-cell lung cancer

- Cetuximab (Erbitux): EGFR antibody.

- Bevacizumab (Avastin): VEGF antibody.

- Trastuzumab (Herceptin): Her-2/neu antibody)

- Tipifarnib (Zarnestra): farnesyltransferase inhibitor.
- Celecoxib (Celebrex): cyclooxygenase-2 inhibitor.
- Bexarotene (Targretin): retinoid X receptor agonist.

Cetuximab (Erbitux)

[Herbst R, *Semin Oncol* **29**(1 Suppl 4): 27–36, 2002]
[Mendelsohn J, *J Clin Oncol* **21**: 2787–2799, 2003]

- Cetuximab is a chimeric immunoglobulin G monoclonal antibody directed against the extracellular ligand binding of HER1.
  - This binding ↓ ligand-induced activation of receptor TK activity, thus inhibiting the effect of HER1 signaling and stimulating receptor internalization.
  - Its antitumor effects are through multiple mechanisms, including inhibition of angiogenesis, promoting apoptosis, and enhancement of immunologic activity.
- Half-life ~ 7 days; the drug can be given weekly as a loading dose of 400 mg/m^2 p.o. followed by a maintenance dose of 250 mg/m^2.
- SIDE-EFFECTS:
  - Acne-like skin rash, asthenia, and allergic reactions.
- Cetuximab can be safely combined with chemotherapy in NSCLC patients.
  - Combination therapies have included platinum-based doublets (with gemcitabine and paclitaxel), and single-agent docetaxel.
    [Kelly K, *Proc Am Soc Clin Oncol* **22**: 644 (abstract 2592), 2003]
    [Kim E, *Proc Am Soc Clin Oncol* **22**: 642 (abstract 2581), 2003]
    [Robert F, *Proc Am Soc Clin Oncol* **22**: 643 (abstract 2587), 2003]
    [Kim E, *Clin Lung Cancer* **6**(Suppl 2): S80–S84, 2004]
- As first-line therapy, cetuximab did <u>not</u> lead to a higher response than chemotherapy alone.
  [Kelly K, *Proc Am Soc Clin Oncol* **22**: 644 (abstract 2592), 2003]
  [Robert F, *Proc Am Soc Clin Oncol* **22**: 643 (abstract 2587), 2003]
- As second-line therapy (cetuximab and docetaxel) showed an ORR of 22.3%, but median survival was only 7.5 months.
  [Kim E, *Proc Am Soc Clin Oncol* **22**: 642 (abstract 2581), 2003]
- A small, phase II, randomized trial compared cisplatin and vinorelbine alone and with cetuximab. The ORR (53.3% vs 32.2%) and disease control rate favored the cetuximab group.
  [Rosell R, *Proc Am Soc Clin Oncol* **23**: 618 (abstract 7012), 2004]

- Phase III trials of chemotherapy with and without cetuximab are ongoing.

Vascular endothelial growth factor

[Ohta Y, *Clin Cancer Res* **2**: 1411–1416, 1996]
[Volm M, *Int J Cancer* **74**: 64–68, 1997]
[Yano T, *Eur J Cancer* **36**: 601–609, 2000]
[Masuya D, *Cancer* **92**: 2628–2638, 2001]
[Minami K, *Lung Cancer* **38**: 51–57, 2002]

- Angiogenesis, the new blood vessel formation from pre-existing vessels, is crucial for tumor growth, development, and metastasis.

- One of the major regulators of neovascularization is VEGF, initially discovered as vascular permeability factor.

- The interaction between VEGF and its TK receptors is an important angiogenesis-regulating process.
  - High levels of VEGF have been associated with poor outcomes in patients with NSCLC.

- Modulation of VEGF-mediated angiogenesis may be approached through the use of antibodies against VEGF protein itself or VEGFR.

Bevacizumab

- Bevacizumab was recently approved by the US Food and Drug Administration for its use in combination with carboplatin and paclitaxel as first-line therapy for patients with metastatic NSCLC, based on the data presented here, especially the ECOG 4599 study.

- Bevacizumab is a recombinant humanized monoclonal antibody to VEGF.
  [Presta L, *Cancer Res* **57**: 4593–4599, 1997]

- Phase I trials showed undetectable VEGF levels when bevacizumab was used at dose of ≥ 3 mg/kg weekly, and no interactions when combined with chemotherapeutic agents.
  [Gordon M, *J Clin Oncol* **19**: 843–850, 2001]
  [Margolin K, *J Clin Oncol* **19**: 851–856, 2001]

- In a randomized, phase II trial, carboplatin and paclitaxel with or without bevacizumab was combined in patients with stage III/IV NSCLC.
  [Johnson D, *J Clin Oncol* **22**: 2184–2191, 2004]

- Two different doses of bevacizumab were studied (7.5 and 15 mg/kg).
- The results from an independent review facility comparing a high vs a low dose of bevacizumab showed:
- RESULTS:
  - Response rate: 40.0% vs 21.9%.
  - Time to progression: 7.0 vs 4.1 months.
  - Median survival: 17.7 vs 11.6 months.
    - all favoring the high-dose bevacizumab group.
- SIDE-EFFECTS:
  - This trial reported an unexpected toxicity, life-threatening hemoptysis (4 deaths) mainly in patients with central tumors and squamous cell histology.
- CONCLUSION:
  - The data suggest that the addition of bevacizumab to carboplatin and paclitaxel resulted in higher response rates, a longer time to disease progression, and improved overall survival.
- LIMITATIONS OF THE STUDY:
  - Potential for investigator bias due to open-label trial design.
  - The fact that 19 of the 32 control patients crossed over to single-agent bevacizumab on disease progression may have impacted on the median survival of this cohort.

- ECOG 4599.
  [Sandler A, N Engl J Med **355**(24): 2542–2550, 2006]
  - Phase III, randomized, placebo-controlled trial.
  - Patients with advanced NSCLC were randomized to bevacizumab (B) 15 mg/kg 3 times weekly vs placebo in combination with carboplatin and paclitaxel (CP).
  - No crossover or patients with squamous cell disease or history of hemoptysis were allowed.
  - RESULTS:
    - 444 patients were assigned to CP and 434 to CPB.
    - Response rate: 10% vs 27% ($p < 0.001$).
    - Progression-free survival (PFS): 4.5 vs 6.4 months ($p < 0.001$).
    - Median survival: 10.2 vs 12.5 months ($p < 0.0075$).
      - all favoring the CPB arm.
  - CONCLUSION:
    - CPB is ECOG's new treatment standard in this patient population.

- Bevacizumab has also been combined with erlotinib.
  [Herbst R, J Clin Oncol **23**: 2544–2555, 2005]
  - The concept of combining specific inhibitors is attractive, and may improve clinical efficacy, with minimal adverse events.

- A phase I/II trial combining these two compounds in patients with advanced non-squamous NSCLC was recently reported.
- RESULTS:
  - PR and stable disease: 20% and 65%, respectively.
  - Median OS of 34 patients treated at the phase 2 dose: 12.6 months.
  - A phase III confirmatory trial is ongoing.

Bevacizumab with other agents

[Fehrenbacher L, *J Clin Oncol* **24**(18 Suppl): abstract 7062, 2006]

- First randomized, phase II study combining erlotinib with docetaxel, pemetrexed, or bevacizumab.
  - PRELIMINARY RESULTS:
    - Possibility of ↑ ORR with the combination of these agents with bevacizumab.

HER2 inhibition

[Kern J, *Cancer Res* **50**: 5184–5187, 1990]

- Trastuzumab is a humanized monoclonal antibody that targets HER-2/neu receptors.

- Once it is activated, it alters several downstream signals, especially the MAPK pathway, and hence causes cell-cycle arrest in the G_0 to G_1 phase.

- HER2 gene amplification is modest in NSCLC, which limits its further development. Her-2/neu overexpression has proven to be an independent, unfavorable prognostic factor in resected patients with NSCLC.

- ECOG 2598
  [Langer C, *J Clin Oncol* **22**: 1180–1187, 2004]
  - A phase II trial of the combination of carboplatin, paclitaxel, and trastuzumab in patients diagnosed with advanced NSCLC.
  - Median overall survival → 10.1 months.
  - 1-year OS: → 42%.
  - CONCLUSIONS:
    - The combination proved to be feasible.
    - OS was similar to historical data using carboplatin and paclitaxel alone.

- Patients with 3+ HER-2/neu expression did well, in contrast to historical data suggesting potential benefit for trastuzumab in this rare subset of NSCLC patients.
- Trastuzumab has also been combined with cisplatin and gemcitabine for the treatment of NSCLC.
  [Zinner R, *Lung Cancer* **44**: 99–110, 2004]
  - 24 chemotherapy-naive patients were enrolled.
  - Stage IIIB or IV NSCLC with either a Her2 score of at least 1+ by immunohistochemical analysis or a serum Her2 shed antigen level of at least 15 ng/ml by enzyme-linked immunosorbent assay.
    - Treatment plan: cisplatin 75 mg/m^2 on day 1, gemcitabine 1250 mg/m^2 on days 1 and 8, and trastuzumab 4 mg/kg on day 1 and 2 mg/kg weekly thereafter on a 21-day cycle for 6 cycles followed by weekly maintenance trastuzumab therapy.
  - RESULTS:
    - 8 (38%) patients had a PR.
    - 1-year survival rate → 62% (13/21).
    - Median time to progression → 36 weeks.
  - CONCLUSIONS:
    - The addition of trastuzumab to cisplatin and gemcitabine was well tolerated.
    - Further study is required to determine whether this combination is superior to chemotherapy alone.
- A multicenter, phase II trial combined cisplatin + gemcitabine with or without trastuzumab in patients with advanced NSCLC who overexpressed or amplified Her-2/neu.
  [Gatzemeier U, *Ann Oncol* **15**: 19–27, 2004]
  - Treatment plan: gemcitabine 1250 mg/m^2 on days 1 and 8, cisplatin 75 mg/m^2 on day 1, and trastuzumab 4 mg/kg i.v. followed by 2 mg/kg i.v. weekly until progression (study group).
  - 619 patients were screened; 103 were eligible.
  - 51 patients were treated with trastuzumab + gemcitabine + cisplatin and 50 with gemcitabine + cisplatin.
  - RESULTS:
    - Efficacy was similar in the trastuzumab and control groups:
      - Response rate: 36% vs 41%.
      - Median time to progression: 6.3 vs 7.2 months.
      - Median PFS: 6.1 vs 7 months.
    - The response rate (83%) and median PFS (8.5 months) appeared relatively good in the 6 trastuzumab-treated patients with HER2 3+ or fluorescence in situ hybridization (FISH) (+) NSCLC.

- CONCLUSIONS:
    - The addition of trastuzumab to gemcitabine + cisplatin was well tolerated.
    - No clinical benefit was observed.
- LIMITATIONS OF THE STUDY:
    - The presence of HER2 3+/FISH (+) (which may benefit most from this therapy) is rare, and this group was too small to provide definitive information.
- Further studies are needed to determine the role of trastuzumab in NSCLC.

Farnesyltransferase inhibitors

[Adjei A, *J Clin Oncol* **21**: 1760–1766, 2003]

- Oncogenic *ras* mutation is found in 40% of NSCLC patients.

- Activating mutations in *ras* proteins translate into constitutive signaling, leading to cell proliferation and inhibition of apoptosis.

- Oncogenic ras protein function is dependent on the location relative to the membrane, a critical step catalyzed by farnesyltransferase, which becomes a therapeutic target of farnesyltransferase inhibitor (FTI) agents.

- As single agents, FTIs have minimal activity in lung cancer.

- Promising results from combining FTIs with conventional chemotherapy warrant further studies using this combination approach for the treatment of NSCLC.
    - The combination of systemic chemotherapy with tipifarnib is under investigation in randomized, phase III trials in patients with advanced NSCLC.
    - In 2004, a phase III trial using lonafarnib was stopped due to lack of efficacy to warrant further enrolment after an interim data analysis.

Cyclooxygenase-2 inhibitors

[Altorki N, *J Clin Oncol* **21**: 2645–2650, 2003]

- Cyclooxygenase-2 (COX-2) is induced by cytokines, growth factors, oncogenes, and tumor promoters.
    - ↑ in NSCLC, especially adenocarcinomas.
- COX-2 catalyzes the rate-limiting step in prostaglandin synthesis and is overexpressed in 70–90% of NSCLC patients.

- In preclinical studies, inhibition of COX-2 was found to enhance the cytotoxic effect of docetaxel.

- Although COX-2 inhibitors were recently removed from the market due to cardiovascular-related events, celecoxib showed ↑ resectability and clinical and pathological response rates in patients with early-stage NSCLC treated with combined chemotherapy (carboplatin + paclitaxel) and celecoxib 400 mg p.o. b.i.d. in the neoadjuvant setting.

- Celecoxib was combined with docetaxel in patients with recurrent disease.
[Csiki I, *Clin Cancer Res* **11**: 6634–6640, 2005]
  - 56 patients were enrolled.
  - Treatment plan: celecoxib 400 mg p.o. twice daily + docetaxel 75 mg/m^2 every 3 weeks to a cohort of patients with recurrent, previously treated NSCLC.
  - Patients first received single-agent celecoxib for 5–10 days to ascertain the effectiveness of COX-2 inhibition, which was determined by measuring pre- and post-celecoxib levels of PGE-M (the major metabolite of prostaglandin E$_2$).
  - RESULTS:
    - ORR → 11%.
    - Median survival → 6 months, similar to that observed with docetaxel alone.
    - Pre-celecoxib urinary PGE-M ↓ from a mean level of 27.2 → 12.2 ng/mg creatinine after 5–10 days of celecoxib ($p = 0.001$).
    - When grouped by quartile, patients with the greatest proportional decline in urinary PGE-M levels had a longer survival than those with no change or an ↑ in PGE-M (14.8 vs 6.3 vs 5.0 months).
  - CONCLUSION:
    - The combination celecoxib + docetaxel at the doses and schedule employed in this study does not improve survival in unselected patients with recurrent, previously treated NSCLC.
    - The survival prolongation in the subset with a marked ↓ in urinary PGE-M levels warrants further investigation of strategies designed to ↓ prostaglandin E$_2$ synthesis in NSCLC.

Bexarotene

[Tontonoz P, *Proc Natl Acad Sci USA* **94**: 237–241, 1997]

- There are two known classes of retinoid receptor: retinoic acid receptors (RARs) and retinoid X receptors (RXRs).

- Bexarotene is a new class of retinoic acid referred as a rexinoid because it is the first RXR-selective retinoid agonist to be studied in humans.

- Bexarotene is approved in the USA for the treatment of cutaneous T-cell lymphoma.

- RXR is unique among the nuclear hormone receptors in that it can dimerize with any of the other nuclear hormone receptors.
    - The formation of those heterodimers affects the function of the gene downstream of retinoic acid response elements (RAREs) by binding DNA.

- Rexinoids affect tumor cells by suppressing proliferation, inducing terminal differentiation, and promoting apoptosis.

- The role of bexarotene in lung cancer was promising based on a multi-institutional, phase I/II trial combining bexarotene with cisplatin and vinorelbine in advanced NSCLC.
  [Khuri F, *J Clin Oncol* **19**: 2626–2637, 2001]
    - Phase I of the study determined the maximum tolerated dose to be 400 mg/m^2 p.o. by day.
    - In phase II of the study, 7/28 (25%) patients reached PR, with 1 having a near CR.
    - Median survival $\rightarrow$ 14 months, with 9/28 patients still alive at > 2 years of follow-up.

- Two phase III, randomized trials have recently shown no survival benefit of bexarotene in combination with chemotherapy when compared with chemotherapy alone.

- Bexarotene + carboplatin + paclitaxel vs carboplatin + paclitaxel in untreated advanced NSCLC.
  [Blumenschein G, *Proc Am Soc Clin Oncol* **23**: 621s (abstract 7001), 2005]
    - 612 NSCLC patients from 6 countries were enrolled.
    - RESULTS:
        - The primary endpoint (OS) was <u>not</u> different ($p = 0.19$).
        - The secondary endpoint (projected 2-year survival) was <u>not</u> different ($p = 0.24$).
        - Severe adverse events were rare and balanced between treatment groups.

- [Jassem J, *Proc Am Soc Clin Oncol* **23**: 627s (abstract 7024), 2005]
    - Randomized, phase III trial comparing bexarotene + cisplatin + vinorelbine vs cisplatin + vinorelbine in untreated advanced NSCLC patients.

- 623 patients from 13 countries were enrolled.
- RESULTS:
  - OS was <u>not</u> different ($p = 0.29$).
  - 2-year survivals were 13.2% and 15.7% for the bexarotene and control groups, respectively ($p = 0.40$).

Vaccine therapy in lung cancer

Introduction

[Raez LE, *Expert Rev Anticancer Ther* **5**(4): 635–644, 2005]
[Raez LE, *Clin Med Res* **3**(4): 221–228, 2005]

- Successful active immunotherapy is expected to be specific and non-toxic.
  - However, the success of immunotherapy in cancer has been sporadic and unpredictable.

- Immunotherapy can be delivered through different mechanisms.
  - Passive immunotherapy (e.g. monoclonal antibodies).
  - Active non-specific immunotherapy (e.g. interferon, interleukin-2 (IL-2), or bacterial adjuvants).
  - Active specific therapy (e.g. vaccination).

- Vaccines may represent an alternative therapy, either as a single modality or in combination with other therapies, by mounting an immune response against tumor cells.
  - Nevertheless, their role in targeting lung cancer has not been studied extensively.

- Recent advances in molecular biology have allowed the identification of new antigens that may become new targets for vaccines from either autologous or allogeneic tumor antigen sources.

General steps of immune tolerance and suppression in cancer

[Disis M, *Clin Lung Cancer* **1**: 294–301, 2000]

- Usually, the first step triggering an immune response is antigen presentation in draining lymph nodes where cytotoxic T-lymphocyte (CTL) undergoes clonal expansion and differentiation.

- The cloned CTLs are released into the blood stream and migrate to the 'diseased' tissue via a complex system of chemotaxis and adhesion receptors.

- There is a failure in immune surveillance of the host, and consequently the malignant cells initiate their proliferation and propagation.
  - In principle, there are two mechanisms of immune evasion with intermediates in between: the priming phase and the effector phase.

- Certain factors, such as TGF-β, interleukin-10 (IL-10), phosphatidyl serine, prostaglandins, and soluble Mic, may inhibit the immune system, hence interfering with adequate priming.
  [Groh V, *Nature* **419**: 734–738, 2002]

Types of vaccine according to their manufacturing process

- Granulocyte–macrophage colony-stimulating factor (GM-CSF) gene transduced tumor cells (e.g. GVAX).

- B7.1 (CD80) used as a co-stimulatory molecule (e.g. ALVAC/B7.1, allogeneic B7.1 vaccine).

- Anti-idiotype vaccine targeting ganglioside GD3 (e.g. BEC2/BCG).

- Peptide-based vaccines (e.g. BLP25, Her-2/neu, WT1, telomerase, and MAGE3).

- Dendritic cell (DC) vaccines pulsated either with autologous or allogeneic antigens (e.g. DCVax).

Tumor vaccines used in lung cancer

BEC2

- BEC2 in combination with bacillus Calmette–Guerin (BCG).
  [Grant S, *Clin Cancer Res* **5**: 1319–1323, 1999]
  - Pilot study; 15 patients were enrolled; study population had both limited- and extensive-disease small-cell lung cancer (SCLC) following a major response to standard chemotherapy.

- Patients received a series of 5 intradermal immunizations consisting of BEC2 2.5 mg plus BCG over a 10-week period.
- RESULTS:
  - All patients developed anti-BEC2 antibodies.
  - 5 patients, including those with the longest relapse-free survival, also developed anti-GD3 antibodies.
  - Median relapse-free survival for patients with extensive disease: 11 months. At the time of publication relapse had not occurred in patients with limited disease (> 47 months).
  - 1/7 patients had a recurrence after a median follow-up → 47 months.

- EORTC 08971, the SILVA Study (Survival in an International Phase III Prospective Randomized Limited Disease Small Cell Lung Cancer Vaccination Study with Adjuvant BEC2 and BCG).
  [Giaccone G, *J Clin Oncol* **23**: 6854–6864, 2005]
  - Phase III, multicenter, randomized trial.
  - 515 patients with a diagnosis of limited-disease SCLC who responded to 4–6 cycles of chemotherapy and thoracic XRT were enrolled.
  - Group I: 258 patients were placed under observation once they had completed chemotherapy and radiation.
  - Group II: 257 patients received BEC2 vaccination once they had completed chemotherapy and radiation.
  - 5 vaccinations (each consisting of eight injections) were planned at weeks 0, 2, 4, 6, and 10.
  - The BEC2 dose was 2.5 mg. BCG was reconstituted in diluent, giving final solutions containing 2.0×10^7, 5.0×10^6, 1.0×10^6, 5.0×10^5, and 1.0×10^5 colony-forming units (cfu) for vaccinations 1–5, respectively.
  - RESULTS:
    - 6 toxic deaths were reported (4 in observation group).
    - Median survival from randomization: 16.4 and 14.3 months in the observation and vaccination groups ($p = 0.28$), respectively.
    - No difference in survival or progression-free survival between observation and vaccination groups.
  - SIDE-EFFECTS:
    - Local skin toxicity, flu-like symptoms, and lethargy.
    - No vaccination-related grade 4 toxicities were observed.
  - CONCLUSION:
    - BEC2/BCG did <u>not</u> confer a survival advantage after a major response to concurrent chemotherapy and radiation therapy (XRT).

GVAX

- Pilot study using GVAX.
  [Salgia R, *J Clin Oncol* **21**: 624–630, 2003]
  - Metastases from 35 patients were resected and processed to single-cell suspension, transfected with a replication-defective adenoviral vector encoding the human GM-CSF gene, irradiated, and cryopreserved.
  - Patients received an intradermal and subcutaneous vaccination weekly for 2 weeks, followed by biweekly vaccination until the vaccine supply was exhausted.
  - RESULTS:
    - 9 patients progressed rapidly and were withdrawn from the study.
    - Vaccinations induced DC, macrophage, granulocyte, and lymphocyte infiltrates in 18/25 patients.
    - Metastatic lesions resected after vaccination revealed tumor necrosis and T-lymphocyte infiltration in 3/6 patients.
    - 5 patients attained stable disease (SD) at 33, 19, 12, 10, and 3 months (all treated at dose level 2).
  - SIDE-EFFECTS:
    - Toxicities were restricted to grade 1–2 local skin reactions.
  - CONCLUSION:
    - Immunization with irradiated autologous non-small-cell lung cancer (NSCLC) cells engineered to secrete GM-CSF elicited antitumor activity in some patients with NSCLC.

- Phase I/II multicenter trial.
  [Nemunaitis J, *J Natl Cancer Inst* **96**: 326–331, 2004]
  [Nemunaitis J, *J Control Release* **91**: 225–231, 2003]
  - Patients with early and advanced stage NSCLC were enrolled.
  - Tumors were harvested from 83 patients, but only 43 patients (10 with early stage I/II and 33 advanced stage III/IV) were vaccinated.
  - RESULTS:
    - 3/33 advanced-stage patients (refractory to standard therapy), 2 of them with BAC, achieved complete response.
    - Duration of the complete responses: > 6 months.
    - Longer median survival (17 months) was observed in patients receiving vaccines secreting GM-CSF at more than 40 ng/24 h per 10^6 cells than in patients receiving vaccines secreting less GM-CSF (median survival 7 months), suggesting a vaccine dose-related survival advantage.
  - SIDE-EFFECTS:
    - The most common toxicity was a local injection-site reaction (93%).

- CONCLUSION:
  - Measurements of immunologic responses were <u>not</u> associated with clinical response or survival.
- LIMITATION OF THE STUDY:
  - The study mixed two populations: early and advanced stage disease.

Vaccines combined with co-stimulatory molecule B7.1 (CD80)

- Phase I trial for patients with advanced (III/IV) NSCLC.
  [Raez L, *J Clin Oncol* **22**: 2800–2807, 2004]
  - Patients were vaccinated using an allogeneic NSCLC tumor cell (AD100) transfected with B7.1 (CD80) and HLA A1 or A2 to study the production of CTLs.
  - 18/19 patients were evaluable; they were vaccinated intradermally once q 2 weeks ×3 (one course) for a maximum of 3 courses.
  - RESULTS:
    - All but 1 patient had a measurable CD8 response after 3 immunizations.
    - The immune response of 6 surviving, clinically responding patients shows that tumor-vaccine-specific CD8 titers continue to be elevated for at least 150 weeks.
    - Overall, 1 patient had a partial response (PR), and 5 had SD.
    - The median survival for all patients was ≥ 18 months, with corresponding estimates of 1-, 2-, and 3-year survivals of 52%, 30%, and 30%, respectively.
    - HLA matching of vaccine, age, sex, race, and pathology did <u>not</u> bear a significant relation to response.
    - As of March 2005, 4/5 patients who achieved SD and the patient who achieved PR were alive, with survivals of: 23, 33, 38, 39, and 52 months, respectively.
    - None of the 13 patients who did not respond to the vaccinations is alive.
  - SIDE-EFFECTS:
    - 4 patients experienced minimal skin erythema.
    - There were no serious adverse events associated with the vaccine.
  - CONCLUSION:
    - B7.1 whole-cell vaccine could induce a moderate to strong CD8 response, with minimal toxicity and good survival, suggesting a clinical benefit from vaccination.

- Phase I trial combining a recombinant poxvirus-based vaccine (ALVAC) and the B7.1.
  [Horig H, *Cancer Immunol Immunother* **49**: 504–514, 2000]
  - 18 patients who had tumor cells expressing carcinoembryonic antigen (CEA) were enrolled.
  - First study to use co-stimulation to enhance the antitumor effect in cancer patients.
  - Three cohorts of 6 patients each were treated with increasing doses of ALVAC-CEA-B7.1 vaccine.
  - Patients who had metastatic adenocarcinoma expressing CEA were vaccinated q 4 weeks for 3 months (only 3 patients had adenocarcinoma of the lung).
  - RESULTS:
    - 3 patients (1 pancreatic cancer, 2 colon cancer) who showed SD underwent repeated vaccination, resulting in augmented CEA-specific T-cell responses.
  - SIDE-EFFECTS:
    - At the highest dose there was no evidence of significant toxicity or autoimmune disorders.
  - CONCLUSIONS:
    - CEA-specific T-cell responses could be sustained with repeated vaccinations.
    - B7.1 may improve the immunologic response to vaccination against tumor-associated antigens.

- This poxvirus-based vaccine is being tested in phase II clinical trials in patients who have cancer cells overexpressing CEA on their cell surface.
  [Ertl H, *Curr Opin Mol Ther* **4**: 601–605, 2002]

Vaccines based on dendritic cells

- Phase I trial to explore the immunologic response to antigen-pulsed DC vaccines in heterogeneous NSCLC patients treated surgically, medically, and by multimodality approaches.
  [Hirschowitz E, *J Clin Oncol* **22**: 2808–2815, 2004]
  [Yannelli J, *Lung Cancer* **47**: 337–350, 2005]
  - 16 individuals with stage IA–IIIB NSCLC treated with surgery, chemoradiation, or multimodality therapy received autologous DC vaccine.
  - Individuals were immunized intradermally twice, 1 month apart.

- RESULTS:
  - Immunologic responses measured by ELISPOT for IFN-γ followed three distinct patterns of reactivity.
    - 5/16 patients showed no clear immunologic response.
    - 5/16 patients showed a tumor-antigen independent response.
    - 5/16 showed an antigen-specific response.
  - Immunologic responses were independent of stage and prior therapy.
  - Favorable and unfavorable clinical outcomes were independent of measured immunologic responses.
- CONCLUSION:
  - DC vaccines were well tolerated and had biologic activity in NSCLC.

- Phase II (preliminary results) trial using DC vaccine transduced with wild-type p53.
  [Gabrilovich D, *J Clin Oncol* **23**: 176s (abstract 2543), 2005]
  - 22 patients with extensive SCLC who attained SD or minor progression after first-line chemotherapy were enrolled.
  - Patients underwent leukapheresis 8 weeks after the last dose of chemotherapy.
  - DCs were then transfected with adenoviral construct containing wild-type p53.
  - Patients received 3 intradermal injections ($2–5 \times 10^6$ p53$^+$ DCs per dose).
  - RESULTS:
    - 5 patients had SD and 17 had progression of disease (most of them within 3 months post-chemotherapy).
    - 11/20 patients had an immunologic response.
    - Those patients who progressed were able to receive second-line chemotherapy.
    - 13 of those patients reached PR ($n = 7$), SD ($n = 2$), and PD ($n = 4$).
  - CONCLUSION:
    - The vaccine was well tolerated and shown to be safe.
    - It induces a substantial immune response, and may sensitize SCLC tumors to subsequent chemotherapy.

- Phase I trial using DCVax.
  [Knutson K, *Curr Opin Mol Ther* **4**: 403–407, 2002]
  - DCVax is an active immunization platform developed by Northwest Biotherapeutics for the potential therapy of several malig-

nancies, including NSCLC, renal, glioblastoma multiforme, and hormone-refractory prostate cancer.
- The DCVax platform is tailored to a specific cancer type using either purified tumor-specific antigen or tumor cell extracts from the patient at the time of surgical resection.
- Ongoing clinical trial.

BLP25 (MUC1) liposomal vaccine

- Phase I trial using MUC1 peptide.
  [Palmer M, *Clin Lung Cancer* 3: 49–57, 2001]
  - 17 patients with stage III/IV NSCLC were enrolled.
  - The safety and tolerability of 2 different vaccine doses (20 and 200 µg) were studied, along with co-administered immunomodulatory doses of cyclophosphamide 300 mg/m² given 3 days prior to vaccination.
  - Patients received subcutaneous injections at weeks 0, 2, 5, and 9.
  - RESULTS:
    - 12 patients completed the vaccination protocol and were evaluable for response. Generation of CTLs against MUC1 (+) tumor cell lines was seen in 5/12 (42%) evaluable patients.
    - No significant humoral or objective anti-tumor responses were seen.
    - 4 (33%) patients achieved SD.
    - Median survival: 5.4 months in the 20 µg group and 14.6 months in the 200 µg group.
  - SIDE-EFFECTS:
    - Hematological toxicity was a clinically insignificant grade 3 lymphopenia (1 patient in each group).
    - Non-hematological toxicities were mild and self-limited.
  - CONCLUSION:
    - BLP25 liposomal vaccine is well tolerated and its major effect is on the cellular immune response in NSCLC.

- A randomized, phase II trial comparing MUC1 peptide-based vaccine vs best supportive care (BSC) as second-line therapy for advanced NSCLC.
  [Butts C, *J Clin Oncol* 23: 6674–6681, 2005]
  - Patients who had stable or responding stage IIIB/IV NSCLC after first-line therapy and ECOG performance status (PS) 0–2 were randomized to either L-BLP25 + BSC or BSC alone.

- Patients in the L-BLP25 group received a single dose of cyclophosphamide 300 mg/m^2 followed by 8 weekly injections of BLP25 1,000 μg.
- Subsequent vaccinations were given at 6-week intervals.
- RESULTS:
  - Median survival: 4.4 months longer for patients randomly assigned to L-BLP25 vaccination (88 patients) compared with the BSC group (83 patients).
  - Adjusted hazard ratio between the two groups was 0.739 ($p = 0.112$).
  - The major effect was seen on stage IIIB vaccinated patients.
  - Median survival has not been reached in this group.
- SIDE-EFFECTS:
  - Most common adverse event was grade 1 flu-like symptoms.
  - Injection-site reactions were described in 45 (51.1%) of 88 patients who received L-BLP25.
- CONCLUSION:
  - L-BLP25 vaccination as maintenance therapy is feasible with minimal toxicity in advanced NSCLC.
  - Although the survival difference between the two groups did not reach statistical significance, a strong trend in 2-year survival in favor of vaccinated patients who had stage IIIB locoregional disease was observed.

WT1 peptide-based vaccine

- Phase I trial using WT1 peptide-based immunotherapy for patients with lung cancer ($n = 10$), breast cancer ($n = 2$), myelodysplastic syndrome ($n = 1$), or acute myeloid leukemia ($n = 13$).
  [Oka Y, *Proc Natl Acad Sci USA* **101**: 13885–13890, 2004]
  - 26 patients received HLA-A restricted, natural, or modified WT1 peptide emulsified with Montanide, an adjuvant administered intradermally at 2-week intervals. Wilm's tumor gene WT1 is over-expressed in leukemias and several solid tumors, including lung cancer.
  - 18 patients completed the WT1 vaccination protocol with 3 or more injections of WT1 peptides.
  - 10 patients had advanced lung cancer.
  - RESULTS:
    - A ↓ in tumor markers caused by WT1 vaccination was seen in 3 patients with lung cancer.
    - These 3 patients received repeated WT1 injections after completion of the initial 3 because of the effectiveness of the vaccine.

- 1 patient has been vaccinated for 2 years without significant side-effects.
- The immunologic response was effective in 3/8 patients with lung cancer who were evaluable for response.
- 2/8 lung cancer patients showed an increase in the frequencies of WT1 peptide–cytoplasmic IFN-γ (+) cells after WT1 vaccination.
- CONCLUSIONS:
  - There was a significant correlation between immunologic and clinical responses.
  - The degree of increase in WT1-specific CTL frequencies may predict clinical response to WT1 vaccination.

Fucosyl GM-1-KLH conjugate-based vaccine

- A phase I trial that utilized a synthetic version of fucosyl GM-1 conjugated to keyhole limpet hemocyanin (KHL).
  [Krug L, *Clin Cancer Res* 10: 6094–6100, 2004]
  - Patients with limited- or extensive-disease SCLC ($n = 16$) who completed initial treatment with chemotherapy (and XRT if indicated) and attained a major response were enrolled.
  - 3 dose levels of fucosyl-GM1-KHL conjugate were studied.
  - QS-21 was used as adjuvant at a dose of 100 µg.
  - Vaccinations were administered intradermally in weeks 1, 2, 3, 4, 8, and 16.
  - RESULTS:
    - 5/6 patients receiving the 30 µg dose and 3/5 patients receiving the 10 µg dose mounted immunoglobulin M responses of 1:80 or greater.
    - Antibodies were confirmed by flow cytometry in 7/8 patients.
    - None of the patients receiving the third dose level had titers above 1:80.
  - SIDE-EFFECTS:
    - No grade 3/4 toxicities were seen.
  - CONCLUSIONS:
    - A dose–response relationship for the doses of 10 and 30 µg is suggested by this trial.
    - A phase II clinical trial using a 'tetravalent' vaccine will combine fucosyl GM-1 at a dose of 30 µg with vaccines against 3 other antigens (GM2, Globo H, and polysialic acid) in patients previously treated for SCLC.

Epidermal-growth-factor-based vaccine

- Two pilot clinical trials, open-label randomized studies, using EGF-based vaccination to treat NSCLC.
  [Gonzalez G, *Ann Oncol* **14**: 461–466, 2003]
  - Data from both pilot studies were analyzed.
  - The studies were intended to compare the safety and immunogenicity of vaccination with an EGF-based vaccine with two different adjuvants (aluminum hydroxide and montanide ISA 51).
  - First trial:
    - 20 patients received an intramuscular vaccine on days 0, 7, 14, 21, and 51.
  - Second trial:
    - 20 patients were randomized and vaccinated as in the first trial but all received a single dose of cyclophosphamide 200 mg/m^2 3 days prior to vaccination.
  - RESULTS:
    - Both pilot trials showed that montanide ↑ the percentage of good antibody responders (GARs).
    - Prevaccination treatment with cyclophosphamide did <u>not</u> provoke an improvement in antibody response.
    - There was a significant ↑ in survival for patients with maintained antibody response.
    - Within the GAR subgroup, the duration of the antibody titers showed an additional correlation with survival.
  - SIDE-EFFECTS:
    - No evidence of severe clinical toxicity was observed.
  - CONCLUSIONS:
    - Vaccination with 5 doses of EGF-based vaccine is safe and immunogenic.
    - Montanide ISA 51 increased the percentage of GARs.
    - There is a direct relationship between anti-EGF antibody titers and the duration of the immune-response with survival time.

- Phase I trial using EGF-based vaccine in advanced NSCLC.
  [Ramos T, *Cancer Biol Ther* **5**(2): 375–379, 2006]
  - 43 patients who received first-line therapy were randomized to receive single or double EGF vaccination.
  - Vaccination was given weekly for 4 weeks, then monthly.
  - RESULTS:
    - 15 (39%) patients developed GAR against EGF.
    - Median survival from randomization: 8.23 months in vaccinated patients.

- Patients who received the double vaccination showed a trend toward ↑ survival compared with patients who received the single dose.
- GARs and patients in whom the serum EGF ↓ below the 168 pg/ml cut-off point had a significantly better survival than did poor responders or patients in whom the EGF levels were <u>not</u> considerably reduced.
- SIDE-EFFECTS:
  - Fever, chills, flushing, nausea, and vomiting.
- CONCLUSIONS:
  - EGF vaccine can mount an immune response against advanced-stage NSCLC.
  - Antibody titers and serum EGF levels appear to correlate with patient survival.

Telomerase peptide-based vaccine

- Phase I/II trial combining the telomerase peptides GV1001 and HR2822.
  [Brunsvig P, J Clin Oncol 23: 185s (abstract 2580), 2005]
  - 26 patients with advanced NSCLC were given intradermal GV1001 (112 or 560 μg) in combination with HR2822 (68.4 μg) and GM-CSF.
- RESULTS:
  - 11/24 evaluable patients had an immune response against GV1001 following the primary vaccination regimen.
  - 2 more patients had an immune response following booster injections.
  - The treatment was well tolerated, with minor side-effects.
  - 1 patient had a complete tumor response and developed GV1001-specific CTL that could be cloned from peripheral blood.
- CONCLUSION:
  - Telomerase vaccination in treatment-resistant NSCLC patients is feasible.
  - It produces a beneficial immune response in 50% of vaccinated patients.

α(1, 3)-Galactosyltransferase-based vaccine

- Phase I trial from the National Cancer Institute.
  [Morris J, J Clin Oncol 23: 187s (abstract 2586), 2005]

- 7 patients with refractory or recurrent NSCLC were treated (as of May 2005).
- 3 irradiated genetically altered human lung cancer cell lines, engineered to express xenotransplantation antigens by retroviral transfer of the murine $\alpha(1, 3)$-galactosyltransferase gene, were injected intradermally (dose escalation per cohort) every 4-weeks ×4.
- Patients received 4 ($n = 4$), 3 ($n = 2$), or 2 vaccinations ($n = 1$).
- RESULTS:
  - 4 patients had SD after > 16 weeks (range 17–28 weeks), and in 3 others there was disease progression.
- SIDE-EFFECTS:
  - Injection-site pain, local skin reaction, fatigue, and hypertension.
- CONCLUSION:
  - The use of this vaccination has proven safe and feasible.

MAGE-3 peptide-based vaccine

- Phase II trial used MAGE-3 protein to treat NSCLC patients in the adjuvant setting.
  [Atanackovic D, *J Immunol* **172**: 3289–3296, 2004]
  - 17 patients with MAGE-3-expressing stage I/II NSCLC were enrolled and analyzed.
  - All patients underwent surgical resection; none had evidence of disease.
  - The first 9 patients received 300 μg of MAGE-3 protein alone; the following 8 patients received MAGE-3 protein combined with AS02B adjuvant.
  - Patients received 4 intradermal injections (protein-alone cohort) or 4 intramuscular injections (protein + adjuvant) at 3-week intervals (days 1, 22, 43, and 64).
  - RESULTS:
    - In the protein-alone cohort 3 patients developed a modest but significant ↑ in antibodies against MAGE-3 protein.
    - In the protein + adjuvant cohort 7/8 patients developed a marked ↑ in antibodies.
    - All 17 patients were examined for CD4$^+$ Th-cell response:
      - Protein-alone cohort: only 1 patient showed a CD4$^+$ T-cell response against MAGE-3.DP4.
      - Protein + adjuvant cohort: all patients were found to have the HLA-DP4 allele, and 4 of them showed a marked increase in CD4$^+$ T-cell responses against MAGE-3.DP4.

- CONCLUSIONS:
  - Vaccination with the recombinant protein of a cancer testis (CT) antigen provides strong antigen-specific CD4$^+$ T-cell help along with antibodies and CD8$^+$ T-cell responses.
  - These results favor an integrated immune response against tumor cell lines.

Her-2/neu-derived peptide based-vaccine

- Phase I trial of Her-2/*neu*-derived peptide in breast and lung cancer patients.
  [Salazar LG, *Clin Cancer Res* **9**: 5559–5565, 2003]
  - A minority of patients immunized with the Her-2/*neu*-derived multipeptide vaccine developed a Her-2/*neu* peptide-specific T-cell immunity or antibody immunity, and none developed Her-2/*neu* protein-specific immunity.
  - This study included only 1 patient with stage III NSCLC.

20

Palliative treatment in lung cancer

- Palliative care is an important part of cancer control.

- The World Health Organization defines palliative care as an approach that improves the quality of life of patients and their families, who are facing the problems associated with life-threatening illness.

- The goal is to prevent or relieve the side-effects and symptoms of cancer and its treatments by means of early identification and immediate assessment and treatment.

- In this chapter we review the basic aspects of the management of anemia, nausea and vomiting, and neutropenic fever, especially in patients with lung cancer.

Anemia and lung cancer

Definition of anemia

[NCCN guidelines 2007: http://www.nccn.org/professionals/default.asp (accessed 8 August 2007)]

- Using a definition of hemoglobin < 12 g/dl, a retrospective review showed that patients receiving radiotherapy for colorectal, lung, and cervical cancer had anemia by the end of treatment in 67%, 63%, and 82% of patients, respectively.

Incidence of anemia

[Groopman JE, *J Natl Cancer Inst* **91**(19): 1616–1634, 1999]

- The incidence and severity of chemotherapy-related anemia depends on a variety of factors, including:
  - Schedule.
  - Intensity of therapy administered.
  - History of prior myelosuppressive chemotherapy.
  - History of radiation therapy (XRT).
  - History of both chemotherapy and XRT.

Other risk factors that ↑ incidence of anemia

[NCCN guidelines 2007: http://www.nccn.org/professionals/default.asp (accessed 8 August 2007)]

- Transfusion within the past 6 months.

- Age.

- Hemoglobin level.

- Anemia has been implicated as a risk factor for poor locoregional tumor control and survival following potentially curative treatment with chemotherapy, XRT, or both, for various solid tumor types, including lung cancer.
  [Crawford J, *Lung Cancer* **38**(Suppl 3): S75–S78, 2002]

- The highest incidence of anemia requiring transfusion occurs in patients with lymphomas, lung tumors, and ovarian or genitourinary tumors, in whom the incidence may be as high as 50–60%.

High-risk chemotherapy agents that impact on anemia in lung cancer

- Platinum-based chemotherapy is the mainstay of the treatment of lung cancer. Patients with this disease commonly experience clinically important decreases in hemoglobin.

- [Okamoto H, *Ann Oncol* **3**: 819–824, 1992]

  In a study of 125 patients with non-small-cell lung cancer (NSCLC), a statistically inverse relationship was found between the accumulated dose of cisplatin and the lowest nadir of hemoglobin ($p = 0.4$).

- Other high-risk agents or combinations include:
  - Paclitaxel + platinum.
  - Paclitaxel + carboplatin.

– The addition of carboplatin or cisplatin to paclitaxel results in a slight ↑ in grade 3 or 4 anemia compared to paclitaxel alone in previously untreated patients with advanced disease.

Impact of anemia and lung cancer

- Fatigue.

- Shortness of breath.

- Diminished ability to perform daily functions.

- Associated with poor prognosis and increased mortality.

- Complicates coexisting disease.

- May compromise efficacy and tolerability of treatment.

Management of anemia

- Treatment is individualized.

- The National Comprehensive Cancer Network (NCCN) provides guidelines on treating cancer-related anemia depending on the severity of the anemia:
  [NCCN guidelines 2007: http://www.nccn.org/professionals/default.asp (accessed 8 August 2007)]
  – Mild: Hgb 10–11 g/dl.
  – Moderate: Hgb 8–10 g/dl.
  – Severe: Hgb < 8 g/dl.

- Treatment should include correction of underlying causes (i.e. simple nutritional deficiencies, underlying infections or inflammatory processes, occult blood loss, or hemolysis).

- Consideration of comorbidities (i.e. renal dysfunction) should be included.

- Management of anemia may depend on whether patient is asymptomatic or symptomatic.
  [NCCN guidelines 2007: http://www.nccn.org/professionals/default.asp (accessed 8 August 2007)]

- Symptomatic treatment includes: red blood cell transfusion, administration of erythropoietin alfa, and/or iron supplementation.

Response assessment

[NCCN guidelines 2007: http://www.nccn.org/professionals/default.asp (accessed 8 August 2007)]

- An initial response assessment distinguishes patients with a response (Hgb increase of 1 g/dl) from those with no response to erythropoietic therapy.

- Patients with a response should be maintained at Hgb 12 g/dl.

- Patients with no response should be assessed at 4 weeks for epoetin alfa and 6 weeks for darbopoietin alfa.

Education of patients related to anemia

- Teach patients to report symptoms of fatigue using a standardized instrument.

- Have patients keep a log of activities or a journal.

- Teach coping strategies (i.e. energy conservation, trying to accept what one cannot change).

Nausea and vomiting

Phases

- Nausea and vomiting can be divided into three different phases:
  - Anticipatory phase, which is a learned response to treatment.
  - Acute phase, which can be further divided into:
    - Acute (0–12 hours post-treatment).
    - Acute late (12–24 hours post-treatment).
  - Delayed phase, which occurs 24 hours after treatment.

Levels of emetic potential of some chemotherapeutic agents

[Hesketh PJ, *Oncologist* 4: 191–196, 1999]

- Level 1 drugs have a negligible risk ($< 10\%$) for emetogenicity.

- Level 2 drugs have a low risk (10–30%) for emetogenicity.

- Level 3 drugs have a moderate risk (30–60%) for emetogenicity.

- Level 4 drugs have a high risk (60–90%) for emetogenicity.

- Level 5 drugs have an extreme risk ($> 90\%$) for emetogenicity.

Managing nausea and vomiting

[Jenns K, *Cancer Nurs* **17**: 488–493, 1994]

- ~ 70–80% of all cancer patients receiving chemotherapy have the potential to experience nausea and vomiting.
- It is considered to be among the most arduous and the most feared consequences of chemotherapy.
  - It is extremely important to control it as it may lead to poor compliance, nutritional deficiency, electrolyte imbalances, and deterioration of self-care.
- Prevention is the key.
  - It is much easier to prevent nausea and vomiting than it is to treat it.
- Some patients may need to use more than one antiemetic agent.
  - The NCCN practice guidelines.
    - Give additional agents from different drug classes until achieving optimal control of nausea and vomiting.

Treating levels of nausea and vomiting

[NCCN guidelines 2007: http://www.nccn.org/professionals/default.asp (accessed 8 August 2007)]
[Gralla RJ, *J Clin Oncol* **17**: 2971–2994, 1999]

- Chemotherapy of high emetogenic risk should be administered with any of the available 5-HT$_3$ receptor antagonists plus a corticosteroid to control acute chemotherapy-induced nausea and vomiting (CINV), followed by treatment with a corticosteroid + metoclopramide, or a corticosteroid + 5-HT$_3$ receptor antagonist, to control delayed CINV.
- Chemotherapy of moderate emetogenic risk should be administered with any of the available 5-HT$_3$ receptor antagonists plus a corticosteroid to control acute CINV, followed by treatment with a corticosteroid alone or with metoclopramide or a 5-HT$_3$ receptor antagonist.
- No routine pretreatment with antiemetics is recommended prior to chemotherapy of low emetogenic risk. Prophylactic treatment with antiemetics is not recommended for patients receiving chemotherapy of minimal emetogenic risk.
- Orally and intravenously administered 5-HT$_3$ receptor antagonists are generally equivalent in efficacy.

- At equipotent doses, commercially available 5-HT$_3$ receptor antagonists do not differ in efficacy or safety and may be selected based on availability and relative cost.

Agents

5-HT3 receptor antagonists

[Heron JF, *Ann Oncol* **5**: 579–584, 1994]

- 5-HT$_3$ receptor antagonists were developed specifically to control emesis associated with highly emetogenic chemotherapy (e.g. cisplatin).
  - These drugs block the amplifying effect of excess 5-HT on vagal nerve fibres and are therefore of specific value in situations where excessive amounts of 5-HT are released from the body's stores (enterochromaffin cells and platelets) following chemotherapy- or XRT-induced damage to the gut mucosa, bowel distension, and renal failure (leaky platelets).

- Granisetron (Kytril).
  - For use in the acute phase.

- Ondansetron (Zofran).
  - For acute phase and radiation-induced nausea.

- Dolasetron (Anzemet).
  - For use in the acute phase.

- Palonosetron (Aloxi).
  - For use in the acute and delayed phases.

Corticosteroids

[Gralla RJ, *J Clin Oncol* **17**: 2971–2994, 1999]
[Gralla RJ, *Semin Oncol* **29**(Suppl 4): 119–124, 2002]

- Corticosteroids play an integral role in the management of delayed CINV.

- Adding corticosteroids to 5-HT$_3$ receptor antagonists has been shown to improve control of acute CINV by 10–20%.

- They may also control CINV from moderately emetogenic chemotherapy when used as a single agent.

- The best example of this class of drugs is dexamethasone (Decadron).

Other agents

Oral neurokinin receptor antagonists (NK1)
[Hesketh PJ, *J Clin Oncol* **17**: 338–343, 1999]
[Navari RM, *N Engl J Med* **340**: 190–195, 1999]

- Aprepitant (Emend).

- A newer class of antiemetics, neurokinin receptor antagonists, has been shown to have antiemetic activity in preventing both acute and delayed CINV when used in conjunction with a 5-HT$_3$ receptor antagonist and a corticosteroid.

Dopamine receptor antagonists
- Prochlorperazine (Compazine).
  - Indicated for mild to moderate nausea and vomiting.
- Metoclopramide (Reglan).
  - Indicated for breakthrough and delayed nausea and vomiting.

Benzodiazepines
- Lorazepam (Ativan).
  - Indicated for breakthrough and anticipatory nausea and vomiting.

Other agents
- Diphenhydramine (Benadryl).

Febrile neutropenia

[NCCN guidelines 2007: http://www.nccn.org/professionals/default.asp (accessed 8 August 2007)]
[Infectious Diseases Society of America guidelines 2002: http://www.idsociety.org/pg/toc.htm (accessed 8 August 2007)]

Fever and neutropenia

- Single temperature reading > 38.3°C (orally) or 101°F.
- < 500 neutrophils/μl, or < 1000 neutrophils/μl and a predicted decline to < 500 neutrophils/μl over the ensuing 48 hours.

Evaluation

- Site-specific history and physical examination.
- Intravenous access device.

- Skin, lungs, and sinus.
- Alimentary canal (mouth, pharynx, esophagus, bowel, rectum).
- Perivaginal/perirectal.

Supplementary and historical information

- Travel.
- Pets, tuberculosis exposure.
- Major comorbid illness.
- Previous blood product administration.
- Recent antibiotic therapy.
- Medications.
- Time since last chemotherapy administration.
- History of prior documented infection.
- Human immunodeficiency virus (HIV) status.

Laboratory and radiological assessments

- Complete blood cell count, comprehensive metabolic panel, urinalysis, chest x-ray, pulse oximetry.

Primary cultures

- Blood ×2 sets.
- Urine (if symptoms, urinary catheter, abnormal urinalysis).
- Site-specific culture.
  - Diarrhea (*Clostridium difficile* assay, enteric pathogen screen).
  - Skin (aspirate/biopsy of skin lesions or wounds).
  - Vascular access cutaneous site if inflammation.
  - Viral cultures.
  - Mucosal or cutaneous vesicular/ulcerated lesions.
  - Throat or nasopharynx during seasonal outbreaks of respiratory viral infections.

Treatment

- Empirical administration of broad-spectrum antibiotics is necessary for febrile neutropenic patients.

- Available diagnostic tests are not sufficiently rapid, sensitive, or specific to identify or exclude the microbial cause of a febrile episode.
- If untreated, these infections may be rapidly fatal in the neutropenic host.
- Although molecular diagnostic technology provides considerable promise, it has added little useful support to the immediate evaluation of febrile neutropenic patients.

Outpatient therapy

- Treatment of carefully selected febrile neutropenic patients with an oral antibiotic alone appears to be feasible for adults at low risk of complications (absolute neutrophil count of > 100 cells/mm^3, normal chest x-ray, duration of neutropenia < 7 days, no i.v. catheter, normal renal and hepatic function, no comorbid complications, resolution of neutropenia expected in < 10 days).
- Patients can be treated with an oral antibiotic.
  - Ciprofloxacin 500 mg p.o. every 8 hours or amoxicillin/clauvinate 500 mg p.o. every 8 hours.
  - For penicillin-allergic patients ciprofloxacin or clindamycin 450 mg p.o. every 6 hours.

Guidelines for therapy

- Initial antibiotic therapy: one of three regimens.
  - If vancomycin is not needed:
    - Monotherapy: ceftazidime or imipenem (cefepime or meropenem), or
    - Duotherapy: aminoglycoside + antipseudomonal β-lactam.
  - If vancomycin is needed (criteria given):
    - Vancomycin + ceftazidime.
- If afebrile within the first 3 days of treatment.
  - If no etiology identified:
    - Low risk (defined): change to oral antibiotic (cefixime or quinolone).
    - High risk (defined): continue same antibiotics.
  - If etiology identified: adjust to most appropriate treatment.
- Persistent fever during the first 3 days of treatment:
  - Reassess on day 4 or 5.
  - If no change: continue antibiotics; consider stopping vancomycin if cultures are negative.

  – If progressive disease: change antibiotics.

- If febrile on days 5–7: add amphotericin B.

Use of colony-stimulating factors in treatment

[Crawford J, *N Engl J Med* **325**: 164–170, 1991]
[NCCN guidelines 2007: http://www.nccn.org/professionals/default.asp (accessed 8 August 2007)]

- Granulocytopenia is a common consequence of many chemotherapy regimens.

- Chemotherapeutic regimens that carry a high risk of febrile neutropenia are:
  – docetaxel + carboplatin (DP).
  – gemcitabine + ifosfamide + vinorelbine (VIG).
  – topitecan + paclitaxel (Top T).
  – cyclophosphamide + doxorubicin + etoposide (CAE).

- Examples of chemotherapeutic regimens that carry an intermediate risk of neutropenia are:
  – cisplatin + paclitaxol (TC).
  – cisplatin + topotecan (TopC).
  – etoposide + carboplatin (EP).

Granulocyte-colony stimulating factor in chemotherapy for small-cell lung cancer

- [Crawford J, *N Engl J Med* **325**: 164–170, 1991]
  - This randomized, double-blind study examined the efficacy of granulocyte-colony stimulating factor (GCSF) in reducing the incidence of neutropenia and febrile neutropenia in patients with small-cell lung cancer.
  - Data from 135 patients who completed 6 cycles of chemotherapy (cyclophosphamide + doxorubicin + etoposide in 21-day cycles ×6 cycles) were analyzed.
  - Patients were randomized to receive either filgrastim (beginning on day 4 and continuing until day 7 of each cycle) or placebo.
  - The primary endpoint of the trial was development of fever and neutropenia (absolute neutrophil count < 0.5, temperature > 38.2°C).
  - RESULTS:
    – In the placebo group, 77% of patients experienced at least 1

episode of fever, whereas only 40% of the GCSF-treated group experienced fever ($p < 0.001$).

- The median duration of an episode of fever for all cycles was 5 days in the placebo group, compared with 4 days in the group that received GCSF.

- CONCLUSION:
  - GCSF use ↓ incidence of febrile neutropenia and neutropenia.

Granulocyte-colony stimulating factor in chemotherapy for breast cancer

- [Vogel C, *J Clin Oncol* **23**: 1178–1184, 2005]
  - Vogel demonstrated that, even in patients with a moderate risk of neutropenia (17%), the use of GCSF is beneficial; for several patients on NSLC chemotherapeutic regimens these can be considered similar circumstances.
  - This randomized, double-blind study was designed to determine whether first- or subsequent-cycle use of pegfilgrastim prevents febrile neutropenia in patients with breast cancer.
  - 928 patients were randomly assigned to either placebo ($n = 465$) or pegfilgrastim ($n = 463$) 6 mg s.c. on day 2 of each 21-day chemotherapy cycle with docetaxel.
  - The primary endpoint was the percentage of patients developing febrile neutropenia.
  - RESULTS:
    - Patients receiving pegfilgrastim, compared with patients receiving placebo, had a lower incidence of febrile neutropenia (1% vs 17%, respectively; $p < 0.001$).
    - First- and subsequent-cycle use of pegfilgrastim, with a moderately myelosuppressive chemotherapy regimen, markedly ↓ febrile neutropenia.

Severe neutropenic events are most frequent during the first cycle of chemotherapy

- In patients with non-Hodgkins lymphoma receiving CHOP, 50% of febrile neutropenic events occurred during the first chemotherapy cycle. [Lyman GH, *Leuk Lymphoma* **44**: 2069–2076, 2003]

- In patients with breast cancer receiving docetaxel, 67% of febrile neutropenic events occurred during the first chemotherapy cycle in the placebo group. [Vogel C, *J Clin Oncol* **23**: 1178–1184, 2005]

- Pegfilgrastim once per cycle vs filgrastim.
  [Holmes FA, *J Clin Oncol* **20**: 727–731, 2002]
  - A multicenter, randomized, double-blind study to determine whether a single injection of pegfilgrastim s.c. 100 μg/kg is as safe as daily filgrastim 5 μg/kg in reducing neutropenia in patients who received 4 cycles of myelosuppressive chemotherapy with doxorubicin and docetaxel.
  - In cycle 1, 11 pegfilgrastim patients (7%) and 18 filgrastim patients (12%) developed febrile neutropenia.
  - The difference between the percentages → 4.9% (two-sided 95% CI, 11.7–1.9).
  - The rate of febrile neutropenia was higher in cycle 1 than in subsequent cycles.
  - RESULTS:
    - Rate of febrile neutropenia in the pegfilgrastim group ≤ rate for the pegfilgrastim group, in all cycles.
    - 9% of patients treated with pegfilgrastim and 18% of patients treated with filgrastim had febrile neutropenia at some point during the study (difference in percentages 9%; two-sided 95% CI, 16.8–1.1%; $p = 0.029$).
    - Pegfilgrastim was associated with a lower overall rate of febrile neutropenia than was filgrastim.

American Society of Clinical Oncology (ASCO) guidelines for implementing GCSF therapy

[Ozer H, *J Clin Oncol* **18**: 3558–3585, 2000]

- These guidelines are outdated.
  - Modifications allow the use of GCSF even in patients with only a moderate risk of neutropenia (17%).

- Routine primary prophylaxis (first-cycle use) in patients with:
  - Expected risk of febrile neutropenia of > 40% (this is being reconsidered).
  - Special circumstances include patients at increased risk of febrile neutropenia.
  - Secondary prophylaxis (subsequent-cycle use).
  - Maintain full dose intensity in chemotherapy-responsive cancers.
  - Treatment of febrile neutropenia.
  - Increased chemotherapy dose intensity.

- Adjunct to bone marrow transplant and peripheral blood stem cell transplant.
- Acute myeloid leukemia/myelodysplastic syndrome.
- ↓ hospitalization and infection.

NCCN guidelines for implementing GCSF therapy

[NCCN, Myeloid Growth Factors Clinical Practice Guidelines in Oncology. Available at: http://www.nccn.org/professionals/physician_gls/f_guidelines.asp (accessed 8 August 2007)]

- The NCCN updated guidelines for the use of GCSF.
  - Patient risk factors, the myelotoxicity of the chemotherapy regimen, and the aim of the treatment (cure, prolongation of survival, or palliation).
  - Before the first cycle of chemotherapy, patients are assessed for the risk of neutropenia and its complications, and are categorized as:
    - High risk: > 20%.
    - Intermediate risk: 10–20%.
    - Low risk: < 10%.
  - The routine use of CSFs in the first and subsequent cycles of chemotherapy is recommended in high-risk patients.
  - The use of CSFs in intermediate-risk patients in the first and subsequent cycles should be considered, with the aim of treatment.
    - If patients are on chemotherapy for palliative reasons, the use of CSFs may not be warranted.
  - The use of CSFs in low-risk patients is not recommended.

- By defining the threshold for high risk and the routine use of CSFs as > 20%, the NCCN guidelines differ from the earlier ASCO guidelines, which define high risk as > 40%.

21

Lung cancer in women

Introduction

[Patel J, JAMA **291**(14): 1763–1768, 2004]
[Parker SL, CA *Cancer J Clin* **47**(1): 5–27, 1997]
[Fu JB, *Chest* **127**(3): 768–777, 2005]

- Carcinoma of the lung is the leading cause of cancer death in both ♂ and ♀, not only in the USA but also throughout the world.
  - It was long thought that this was a disease which primarily affected ♂.
  - This perception started to change when lung cancer incidence in ♀ began to ↑ and, ultimately, surpassed breast cancer in 1987 as the leading cause of cancer deaths in ♀.

- In 2001, a report of the Surgeon General titled *Women and Smoking* noted that the 600% ↑ in the death rate from lung cancer in ♀ was a 'full-blown epidemic'.

- ♀ started smoking in significant numbers during and following World War II.

- The lung cancer death rate for ♀ rose slowly from about 2.5 cases per 100,000 in 1930 to about 5 cases per 100,000 in 1960.
  - Since 1960 the lung cancer death rate has ↑ rapidly and steadily, and in 1990 it was over 30 per 100,000 ♀.

- Although the prevalence of cigarette smoking in ♀ ↓, it did not do so as much as that in ♂.
  - Beliefs such that smoking helps control weight have motivated many young ♀ to smoke.

– > 20 million American ♀ smoke and there is now a large proportion of teenage girls who use tobacco products.

Lung cancer and smoking in women

[Patel J, *J Clin Oncol* **23**(14): 3212–3218, 2005]
[Fu JB, *Chest* **127**(3): 768–777, 2005]
[Baldini EH, *Chest* **112**(4 Suppl): 229s–234s, 1997]

- In 2003, 44% of the 157,200 lung cancer deaths were reported to be in ♀.
  - There were actually more ♀ dying from lung cancer than from breast, ovarian, and uterine cancer combined.

- The highest frequency of smoking is seen among American Indian and Alaska Native ♀, the frequency being intermediate in Caucasian and African American ♀.
  - The lowest incidence is among Hispanic, Asian, or Pacific Islander ♀.

- Smoking prevalence is nearly ×3 ↑ among ♀ with 9–11 years of education compared with that in ♀ with ≥ 16 years of education.
  - According to the US Centers for Disease Control and Prevention, at least 500,000 teenage girls use tobacco products.

- Despite ↑ knowledge of the adverse health and teratogenic effects of smoking, the incidence of smoking during pregnancy has ↓ only slightly.
  - Of the 4 million ♀ who deliver babies each year, ~ 1 million of them smoke during pregnancy.

- ♀ who smoke appear to have a greater risk of developing:
  - Small-cell lung cancer (SCLC) than ♂ who smoke.
  - Adenocarcinoma of the lung than ♂ smokers.
  - Evidence which suggests a possible role of exogenous and endogenous estrogens.

Risk factors for female smokers

[Buch S, *Mol Carcinog* **42**(4): 222–228, 2005]
[Shriver SP, *J Natl Cancer Inst* **92**(1): 24–33, 2000]
[Pope M, *J Gend Specif Med* **2**(6): 45–51, 1999]

- The risk of developing lung cancer ↑ with the quantity, duration, and intensity of smoking. The risk of dying of lung cancer is 20 times higher among ♀ who smoke ≥ 2 packs of cigarettes per day than among ♀ who do not smoke.

- ♀ smokers face some unique additional risks:
  - Menstrual irregularities and earlier menopause.
  - Infertility.
  - Bone-thinning osteoporosis.
  - Arthritis.
  - Cervical cancer.
  - Thrombosis, if using birth control pills.
  - If pregnant, low birth weight, stillbirths, miscarriages, and sudden infant death syndrome.

- Findings suggest that having two gene mutations, XPD and cyclin D1, ↑ lung cancer risks in smokers.
  - XPD is involved in repairing everyday damage that occurs naturally when cells divide.
  - Damage to this gene causes genetic damage that accumulates in the cell.
  - Cyclin D1 plays a role in regulating the life cycle of the cell.
  - Damage to this gene allows cells to divide and proliferate abnormally.

- A gene called the gastrin-releasing peptide receptor (GRPR) is linked with abnormal cell growth and is much more active in ♀ than ♂.
  - Because the gene is found on the X chromosome, it may explain why ♀ smokers are ×2 more likely to develop lung cancer than ♂ smokers.
  - This gene prompts cells to link up with the GPR hormone, and that link in turn causes abnormal cell growth that can lead to lung cancer.

Reducing prevalence of smoking among women

[Jodi W, *J Commun Health* **31**(3): 225–248, 2006]

- Currently, < 20% of the states in the USA require schools to offer smoking-prevention services.
  - For example, in Florida in 1998 a campaign by teenagers educating other teens ↓ smoking by middle-school girls from 18.1% to 10.9%.

Other factors linked to women with lung cancer

Family history

[Schwartz AG, *Am J Epidemiol* **144**(6): 554–562, 1996]
[Osann KE, *Cancer Res* **51**: 4893–4897, 1991]

- It is well known that patients with lung cancer have a higher number of relatives with lung cancer than control subjects.
  - The simplest explanation is the clustering of cigarette smokers within families.
  - Perhaps there is an ↑ risk of lung cancer regardless of family smoking history.

- The ↑ risk associated with smoking in ♀.
  [Horwitz RI, *Arch Intern Med* **148**: 2609–2612, 1988]
  - Odds ratios (ORs) for developing lung cancer in ♀ non-smokers with a family history of lung cancer, in ♀ smokers, and in ♀ smokers with a family history of lung cancer are 2.8, 11.3, and 30, respectively.

- A history of prior lung disease.
  [Wu AH, *Am J Epidemiol* **141**(11): 1023–1032, 1995]
  [Alavanja MC, *Am J Epidemiol* **136**: 623–632, 1992]
  - Another known risk factor for ♂ was associated with a relative risk (RR) of developing lung cancer of 1.2 and 1.56 in two case–control studies limited to ♀.

Diet

[Smith-Warner SA, *Int J Cancer* **107**(6): 1001–1011, 2003]
[The Alpha-Tocopherol, Beta-Carotene Cancer Prevention Study Group, *N Engl J Med* **330**: 1029–1035, 1994]
[Menkes MS, *N Engl J Med* **315**: 1250–1254, 1986]
[Steinmetz KA, *Cancer Res* **53**: 536–543, 1993]

- Several publications have mentioned that a higher dietary intake of fruits and vegetables was associated with ↓ risk of lung cancer.

- Case–control studies.
  [Seow A, *Int J Cancer* **97**: 365–371, 2002]
  [Zhong L, *Epidemiology* **12**: 695–700, 2001]
  - Fruit intake and the use of soy in Chinese ♀ provided a protective effect against lung cancer.
  - The same protective effect was observed with the consumption of green tea in a population-based, case–control study.

[Speizer FE, *Cancer Causes Control* **10**: 475–482, 1999]
[Michaud DS, *Am J Clin Nutr* **72**: 990–997, 2000]
- ♀ who consumed < 5 carrots/week had a RR of 0.4 (95% CI, 0.2–0.8) compared with the risk for ♀ who had not consumed carrots.

- A 10-year follow-up of a cohort of ♂ in the Health Professionals Follow-up Study and a 12-year follow-up period of a cohort of ♀ in the Nurses Health Study.
  - New lung cancers were diagnosed in 275/46,924 ♂ and 519/77,283 ♀.

- The risk of lung cancer was significantly ↓ in those who had consumed a variety of carotenoids for a maximum protective period of 4–8 years even after adjusting for residual confounding from smoking (RR +0.68; 95% CI, 0.49–0.94, for the highest compared with the lowest total carotenoid intake).
  - The association was stronger in ♀ than in ♂.
  - Among ♀ never-smokers, a significant 63% lower risk was noted.

- Due to the lack of consistent, reproducible, and strong evidence, many researchers believe that the relationship between diet and vitamins and lung carcinogenesis is unsolved.

Ethnic and racial differences

[Haiman CA, *N Engl J Med* **354**(4): 333–342, 2006]

- The age-adjusted lung cancer incidence in African American ♀ was 10–20% higher than in white ♀.
  - Since 1975 the ↑ has been 120% in African American and 89% in white ♀.
  - Since 1985 the incidence rates have continued to ↑ at an average annual rate of 2.4% for African American and 2.2% for white ♀.

- The Multiethnic Cohort Study showed that among cigarette smokers:
  - African Americans and Native Hawaiians are more susceptible to lung cancer than whites, Japanese Americans, and Hispanics.

Human papilloma virus infection

[Hennig EM, *Acta Oncol* **38**: 639–647, 1999]
[Cheng Y-W, *Cancer Res* **61**: 2799–2803, 2001]
[Tsuhako K, *J Clin Pathol* **51**: 741–749, 1998]
[Kaya H, *Pathologica* **93**: 531–534, 2001]
[Gorgoulis VG, *Hum Pathol* **30**: 274–283, 1999]

- Human papilloma virus (HPV) DNA was detected, utilizing polymerase chain reaction (PCR) and in situ hybridization, in the tumors of 49% of ♀ with lung cancer who also had a history of high-grade (grade 3) chemotherapy-induced nausea and vomiting.

- A Taiwanese study revealed the presence of HPV DNA (types 16 and 18) in the cancer cells of non-smoking ♀ with lung cancer.
  - Interestingly, HPV infection seems to be more associated with squamous cell carcinoma of the lung.
- There is far from universal agreement that HPV is an etiologic agent in lung cancer.
  - An analysis of paraffin-embedded tissue from 32 squamous bronchial carcinomas and 15 cervical cancers, utilizing both in situ hybridization and PCR techniques, was (–) for HPV in the lung cancer cases, but (+) for 12/15 cervical cancer cases.

Epidermal growth factor receptor and lung cancer

[Fukuoka M, *J Clin Oncol* **21**: 2237–2246, 2003]
[Kris MG, *JAMA* **290**: 2149–2158, 2003]
[Perez-Soler R, *J Clin Oncol* **22**: 3238–3247, 2004]
[Tsao MS, *N Engl J Med* **353**: 133–144, 2005]

- Early in the development of tyrosine kinase inhibitors, several phase II studies showed that ♀ sex, adenocarcinoma, Asian origin, and never having smoked are all associated with responsiveness of non-small-cell lung cancer (NSCLC) to erlotinib or gefitinib.
- An analysis found epidermal growth factor receptor (EGFR) mutations in 16/119 tumors, with a predominance of mutations in 15/28 (28%) specimens from Japan, as compared with 1/61 (2%) specimens from the USA.
  [Paez J, *Science* **304**: 1497–1500, 2004]
  - The mutations were much more common in ♀ (9/45; 20%) than in ♂ (7/74; 9%).
  - The highest fraction of EGFR mutations was observed in Japanese ♀ with adenocarcinoma (8/14; 57%).
- Another study, mutational analysis of the EGFR coding sequence, was done on 101 fresh-frozen lung tumor tissues.
  [Huang S, *Clin Cancer Res* **10**: 8195–8203, 2004]
  - Among the 101 patients, 39% carried EGFR mutations within the tumor.
  - Of the 69 patients with adenocarcinoma, 56% had at least one mutation in exons 18–21 of the EGFR gene.
  - There was no significant difference in the EGFR mutation rate between ♂ (18/33; 54.5%) and ♀ (20/36; 55.5%) with adenocarcinoma, and the mutation patterns were also similar in the two groups.

Hormonal influences in women with lung cancer

[Canver CC, *J Thorac Cardiovasc Surg* **108**: 153–157, 1994]
[Cagle PT, *Cancer Res* **50**: 6632–6635, 1990]
[Ollayos CW, *Arch Pathol Lab Med* **118**: 630–632, 1994]
[Matsuda S, *Proc Natl Acad Sci USA* **90**: 10803–10807, 1993]
[Stabile LP, *Cancer Res* **62**: 2141–2150, 2002]

- It has been observed that lung cancer specimens from ♀ are more likely to express estrogen receptors than are those from ♂. Immuno-histochemistry detects expression of the estrogen receptor in 7–97% of cases.

- Results from these investigators are thus far inconsistent.

- Estrogen receptors have also been found in the different histological subtypes of NSCLC.

- Researchers have shown that β-estradiol produced a proliferative response in vitro in both normal lung fibroblasts and cultured NSCLC tumor cells. In vitro and in vivo studies have shown that β-estradiol stimulated growth of the NSCLC tumor line, H23, grown as tumor xenografts in SCID mice.

[Taioli E, *J Natl Cancer Inst* **86**: 869–870, 1994]
- Using case–control data this study demonstrated how menopause prior to age 40 years was associated with a ↓ in lung cancer (OR = 0.3).

- The use of exogenous estrogens was also associated with a modest ↑ risk of lung cancer (OR = 1.7).
  - Smoking was also found to have a possible interaction with estrogen replacement and the development of adenocarcinoma of the lung (OR = 32).

[Blackman J, *Pharmacoepidemiol Drug Safety* **11**: 561–567, 2002]
- Another trial using a similar method of analysis, among ♀ who used estrogen replacement therapy for a minimum of 3 months.
  - OR = 1.0 for the development of lung cancer.

- Using a case–control design.
  [Schabath M, *Clin Cancer Res* **10**: 113–123, 2004]
  - Evaluated the association between hormone replacement therapy and the risk of lung cancer in almost 500 ♀ with lung cancer and 519 age-matched controls.
  - The use of hormone replacement therapy was associated with a 34% overall ↓ in lung cancer risk after controlling for age, menopausal status, ethnicity, body mass index, and tobacco exposure.

- However, this study did not thoroughly assess the dose or the duration of estrogen therapy, thereby leaving much doubt about the results.

The role of genetics

[Haugen A, *Carcinogenesis* **23**: 227–229, 2002]
[Mollerup S, *Cancer Res* **59**: 3317–3320, 1999]
[Cheng YW, *Environ Mol Mutagen* **37**: 304–310, 2001]

- It is believed that DNA adducts are important in lung tumorigenesis because the extent of DNA adduct formation depends on the balance between the rates of oxidation of the carcinogenic compounds in tobacco smoke, DNA repair capacity, and the rates of detoxification of the reactive products via conjugation.
  - Moreover, the level of DNA adduct in the lung could be an exposure marker to carcinogens, as well as a useful factor to be considered for lung cancer susceptibility.

- These DNA adducts have been found in higher levels in ♀ than in ♂ smokers when compared by pack-years of tobacco smoking.

- Furthermore, DNA adducts have been found in higher levels in a series of non-smoking Taiwanese ♀ than non-smoking ♂, and it may reflect the environmental exposure to carcinogens in the Asian population.
  - A higher frequency of a specific mutation (G:C—T:A) in the *p53* gene and a higher average level of DNA adduct were found in lung tumors from both ♂ and ♀.

- *K-ras*, a proto-oncogene of the *Ras* family, has been found in lung cancer, and its incidence is ×3 ↑ ♀ than ♂.
  [Nelson HH, *J Natl Cancer Inst* **91**: 2032–2038, 1999]
  [Ahrendt SA, *Cancer* **92**: 1525–1530, 2001]
  [Wang YC, *J Cancer Res Clin Oncol* **124**(9): 517–522, 1998]

- In ♀ smokers, *K-ras* mutations have been found more frequently in NSCLC than in ♂ smokers.

- *K-ras* oncogene activation by point mutation occurs in about 30% of lung adenocarcinoma in Caucasians.
  - However, *K-ras* gene mutation was found in 13–19% of lung adenocarcinomas in Asian ♂ and it was not present in ♀ patients.
  - An explanation for these findings is the fact that point mutation in *K-ras* is secondary to the mutagenic effect of tobacco, and most Chinese ♀ are non-smokers.

- *CYP1A1* gene.
  [McLemore TL, *J Natl Cancer Inst* **82**: 1333–1339, 1990]
  - Another important gene, which encodes an enzyme for the metabolism of carcinogenic polycyclic aromatic hydrocarbons.
  - Overexpressed in lung tumors from ♀ smokers compared with ♂ smokers.

- The study concluded that the *GSTM1* null genotype effect is higher in ♀ smokers, which is consistent with other reports in which ♀ are at ↑ risk of lung tumorigenesis than ♂ at equal tobacco exposure, especially when both *CYP1A1* and *GSTM1* gene polymorphism are combined.
  [Dresler C, *Lung Cancer* **30**: 153–160, 2000]

- Other prognostic markers in lung cancer, such as *ERCC1, Her-2 neu,* and *RXRβ*, appeared to be sex specific.
  [Dannenberg K, *Proc Am Soc Clin Oncol* **22**: 619s, 2004]

- High levels of these receptors predicted a better survival in ♀, but not in ♂.
  - Conversely, high ornithine decarboxylase expression and a low level of cyclooxygenase-2 predicted better survival in ♂, but not in ♀.

- Although the study included a small number of patients, it emphasized important differences between the genders when analyzing risk factors and predictive and prognostic markers.

Prognosis of women with lung cancer

- In general, ♀ with lung cancer respond better to therapy than ♂ patients, regardless of histology, stage, and modality of treatment.
  - Because the incidence of lung cancer is higher in ♀ and it has steadily ↑ in recent years, lung cancer in ♀ has gained the attention of researchers.

- The Surveillance, Epidemiology and End Results (SEER) database of 31,226 lung cancer patients analyzed several variables in terms of prognosis.
  [Ramalingam S, *Am J Clin Oncol* **6**: 651–657, 1998]
  - ♀ sex was identified as a favorable prognostic factor.

[Radzikowska E, *Ann Oncol* **13**: 1087–1093, 2002]
- ♀ patients had better prognosis than ♂ with lung cancer.

- Regarding the treatment modality used, ♀ did better than ♂, and ♀ were younger, adenocarcinoma and SCLC were the most common histological subtypes, and more ♀ than ♂ patients were non-smokers.

- In a multivariate analysis of this population-based study of 20,561 cases of lung cancer, the RR of death was significantly higher in ♂ (RR = 1.15; $p < 0.001$).

[Albain KS, *J Clin Oncol* **13**: 1880–1992, 1995]
[Graham MV, *Int J Radiat Oncol Biol Phys* **33**: 993–1000, 1995]
[Kirsh MM, *Ann Thorac Surg* **34**: 34–39, 1982]
[Bignall JR, *Lancet* **2**: 60–62, 1972]
[Harley HRS, *Thorax* **31**: 254–264, 1976]

- The available data in terms of outcome based on gender are also conflicting.
  - Some reports have suggested that ♀ had better outcome when surgery, concurrent chemoradiation, or triple modality (surgery, chemotherapy, and radiation) are used.

- Other surgical studies have shown better outcome in ♂ affected by lung cancer.

[Spiegelman D, *J Clin Oncol* **7**: 344–354, 1989]
[Skarin AT, *Chest* **103**: 440S–444S, 1993]
[Sagman U, *J Clin Oncol* **9**: 1639–1649, 1991]
[Albain KS, *J Clin Oncol* **8**: 1563–1574, 1990]
[Lassen U, *J Clin Oncol* **13**(5): 1215–1220, 1995]

- In SCLC series, a multivariate analysis from the Cancer and Leukemia Group B showed a significantly better response and survival rates for ♀ compared with their ♂ counterparts.

- Some studies have found ♀ gender to be a favorable prognostic factor in terms of SCLC survival.
  - However, these observations have not been uniformly confirmed.

[Fukuoka M, *J Clin Oncol* **21**: 2237–2246, 2003]
[Kris MG, *JAMA* **290**: 2149–2158, 2003]

- Although ♀ gender has been associated with longer survival in lung cancer, it has not been correlated with radiographic response to chemotherapy.
  - Nonetheless, a clinical trial using an EGFR inhibitor, gefinitib, showed a better radiographic response in ♀ patients and in the adenocarcinoma histological type.

- Clearly, this observation of improved survival in ♀ with lung cancer may have implications for the future design and interpretation of clinical trials.

Index